Letters from Martin Felt's clients:

'Martin Felt is meticulous, original, brilliant and, in my experience, right!'

Luther Davis, playwright, author of *Grand Hotel* and *Kismet*

'For eighteen months before seeing Martin Felt I had severe irritable bowel syndrome and acute gastritis, having been diagnosed with Cushings Syndrome back in 1980.

'After analysis and instruction from Martin, I was able to pin down several foods that I am allergic to or unable to digest. Nine months later I look five years younger have more energy and I am gradually extending my diet. I continue to abide by my individual Felt Formula.'

Sheila Kendall-Edgecombe, Devon

'As a result of treatment with Martin Felt my complexion has improved, my cellulite has literally melted away and I have lost weight. I've started winning more squash matches, my stomach, teeth and skin problems have disappeared. There was such a noticeable improvement that people regularly ask me what my secret is. That's how I'm able to recommend people to Martin without trying.

'The whole experience has been a real education for me and although I cheat occasionally I now know how to eat.

Carole Golten (37 but feel 27), London

'Almost immediately after changing my diet as directed by Mr Felt I began to feel a difference – I lost 2 stones in weight in less than a month and my migraine headaches stopped altogether. My memory and concentration both became much better.'

Mrs G.T., London

'I went to Martin Felt for depression problems. I'd been feeling this way for many years. He told me what foods to stay away from and gave me a food plan to follow. He also gave me vitamins and herbs to take. It took me about 85 hours to really start feeling well.

I feel like a totally new and healthy person. My friends have even noticed the change. Martin Felt is really on to something that could help everyone.'

Jennifer Bassey, actress and writer

'I have now finished all my cancer treatments and thanks to Martin Felt I do not seem to have any side effects so far. I am following his programme and notice an improvement in myself.'

Mrs L., Cardiff (treated before undergoing chemotherapy)

'I first consulted Martin Felt because I was having unpleasant reactions to eating carbohydrate. Three weeks after the first consultation, I felt so much better. I am eating a well-balanced diet and carbohydrates are no problem to me – I do so enjoy tucking into all the foods I had avoided over the previous 5 years as they caused severe headaches, emotional upsets and fatigue, etc. I am deeply grateful to Martin Felt and his system of nutrition. So simple, so effective.'

Mrs Gina Van der Molen, Croydon

'When I went to see Martin Felt in November 1992, I was gaining weight and suffering chronic acid indigestion. My indigestion disappeared instantly. I lost a stone in weight in 3 months. I like to eat well and I have been able to keep to Martin's regime without feeling seriously deprived.'

John S., London

'In October 1990 I was told that I had a form of lymphatic cancer called Hodgkin's Disease. From February 1991 until January 1992 I was treated with chemotherapy and radiotherapy by one of the world's experts on this condition. Finally I was declared all clear. Unfortunately my blood readings continued to be unstable, indicating a continuing unhappy liver. None the less, the liver and cancer experts released me.

'My energy did not return and in August 1992 I suddenly broke out in a rash beginning on my ears and spreading to my neck, shoulders, face and finally upper arms. My nervous system could not endlessly sustain the unabated itching; life was becoming unbearable. Neither the liver nor the cancer expert believed it had anything to do with them nor their treatment of me. No one seemed interested.

'I first visited Mr Felt in October 1992. He asked me many questions regarding my health history, my emotional and family life and finally practical questions about my current diet and physical habits. During this first encounter with him he explained his system, how the drugs and treatment in general had left my body in a weakened state, how my psychological and social history had informed both the original illness and my current state.

'I followed his regimen carefully and began to gain relief very quickly. By Christmas I was 95 per cent better. I still rely upon his advice and it is clear that my body is slowly readjusting itself and ridding itself of the drugs.

'It is my opinion that Mr Felt's system fills a yawning gap in the practice of contemporary medicine.'

Mr R.G., London

The experts' opinions:

'Within minutes of filling in Martin Felt's questionnaire he had produced a disturbingly accurate physical, emotional, even psychological breakdown of me – I was stunned as he outlined my whole persona. I am naturally lazy when it comes to making changes for the sake of health and fitness, and I left impressed at how simple the system is, and just how easily obtainable a feeling of enhanced well-being can be.'

Newby Hands, Daily Mail

'Having suffered fanatical cravings for kidneys and chocolate throughout my pregnancy, I have adopted Felt's recommended diet. He promised that my craving would diminish within 96 hours and that in 3 weeks they should be eliminated. Not only is he as good as his promise, but I feel vigorous for the first time in 6 months.'

Antonia Kirwan-Taylor, Vogue

'It is a seemingly simplistic set of questions which uncannily unfolds into a complex analysis revealing the person's present state of health, and the causes, emotional condition and even any past traumas experienced. As most of his clients discover, it is precise and accurate, it can unveil things about yourself you didn't even realise and offer almost immediate solutions.'

Philippa McKinley, Here's Health

'In 20 years of exploring nutritional systems I have never come across anything so powerful, finely tuned and effective.'

Leslie Kenton, Mirabella

Martin Felt runs a private practice in London where people consult him for every type of health concern from clinically healthy people who want to achieve optimal fitness to those with serious diagnosed diseases.

Over the past twenty years he has pioneered a unique method of treating the body, mind and spirit in a truly holistic fashion. *Eat Yourself Fit with The Felt Formula* offers a simple and concise method for self care.

If after reading the book you would like an in-depth personal consultation with Martin Felt please write, enclosing a stamped self-addressed envelope, to the following address:

> Martin Felt
> c/o Limelight Management
> 9 Coptic Street
> London WC1A 1NH

EAT YOURSELF FIT WITH THE WITH THE FELT FORMULA

Martin Felt

HEADLINE

First published in 1994
by HEADLINE BOOK PUBLISHING

10 9 8 7 6 5 4 3 2 1

Felt, Martin
    Eat Yourself Fit with the Felt Formula
    I. Title
    613.2

    ISBN 0-7472-0943-X (hardback)
    ISBN 0 7472 7847 4 (softback)

Typeset by
Letterpart Limited, Reigate, Surrey

Printed and bound in Great Britain by
Mackays of Chatham PLC, Chatham, Kent

HEADLINE BOOK PUBLISHING
A division of Hodder Headline PLC
Headline House
79 Great Titchfield Street
London W1P 7FN

In 1990, while contemplating writing THE FELT FORMULA I came across the *Complete Works of William Blake* and found a quotation that dazzled me and gave me the hope that I could successfully complete this book.

> Trembling I sit day and night; my friends are astonished at me
> Yet they forgive my wanderings, I rest not from my great task –
> To open the eternal worlds, to open the immortal eyes
> Of man inwards into the worlds of thought – into Eternity
> Ever expanding in the bosom of God, the human imagination.
> O Saviour, pour upon me thy spirit of meekness & love;
> Annihilate the selfhood in me, be thou all my life.
> Guide thou my hand which trembles exceedingly upon the
>   Rock of Ages.

Jerusalem, Emanation of the Giant Albion,
16-24, William Blake

Contents

Acknowledgements   xi
How to use this book   xii
Foreword by Norma Williams MD (USA) MBBS LRCP MRCS (UK)   xiii
Introduction   xv

Part One
1. The Global View   3
2. Your Health in the Balance   13
3. What is Disease?   26
4. Balance and Diet   35

Part Two
The Questionnaire   55

Part Three
The Glands and Organs
Group 1	The Immune System	65
Group 2	The Heart and the Cardiovascular System	76
Group 3	The Colon and the Elimination System	83
Group 4	The Digestive System	88
Group 5	The Sinus, Ears, Nose and Throat	92
Group 6	The Liver and Gall Bladder	96
Group 7	The Lungs and the Respiratory System	101
Group 8	The Sex Organs and the Reproductive System	105
Group 9	The Skeletal and Muscular Systems	111
Group 10	The Thyroid Gland and Metabolism	115
Group 11	The Veins, Arteries and Capillaries of the Circulatory System	118
Group 12	The Brain and the Central Nervous System	122

Group 13	The Adrenal Glands and the Energy System	126
Group 14	The Mind-Body Connection	130
Group 15	The Sensory Mechanism (Sight, Touch, Taste, Smell and Hearing)	133
Group 16	The Kidneys, Bladder, Urethra and Prostate	136
Group 17/18	The Male/Female Hormone Balance and the Endrocrine System	139
Group 19	The Skin and the Excretory System	143
Group 20	The Pancreas and the Energy System	147
Group 21	Water Balance and the Master Hormone Regulator	150
Group 22	The Calcium Controller or Parathyroid	154
Group 23	The Auto-immune System and the Spleen	156
Group 24	The Lymphatic System	160

Part Four

The Five Phases	168
The Five Phase Food Chart	170
The Healing Qualities of Food	174
The Use of Supplements: Vitamins and Minerals	187
Specific Illness Reference List	207
Resource Guide	212
Bibliography	220

Acknowledgements

I would like to thank my agent Fiona Lindsay of Limelight Management for suggesting that I write this book and giving me her unfailing encouragement; Eleanor Lines who assisted me so ably as my personal editor. I have benefited greatly from my association with Headline Book Publishing under the guidance of Anna Powell and the additional editing of Katherine Pate.

I acknowledge my Mentor Dr R. P. Kaushik who inspired me on to the path of nutritional discovery. I acknowledge Vickie Giles whose continual support helped me to keep writing; Rabbi Laurence Alpern whose friendship over the years kept me smiling and laughing when I had lots of doubts about myself and my abilities; my friend Paul Cox who was always 'on the other end of the telephone' to talk and encourage me through the blocks.

I would like to thank all my clients who made the greatest contribution to this book; the Restaurant Gran Paradiso who fed me beautiful foods when I needed to eat during my nights of writing and lastly my personal typist, Lucy, whose conversation between typing made me howl with laughter, lightening the load.

How to use this book

The chapters in Part One describe how the pollution in the atmosphere and the high stress levels of today's societies have affected the chemical balances in our bodies. By discovering your individual Felt Formula you can bring your body back into balance by eating foods to reflect your body's needs.

Part Two is the questionnaire which will interpret your symptoms. Your score indicates your personal stress level and directs you to two groups in Part Three that are relevant to you.

Turn to the two specific groups in Part Three for your psychological and physical profile. Here you will find specific advice on how to resolve the problems you are having through diet, nutritional supplements and homeopathic remedies.

Refer to Part Four for lists of foods you should increase or decrease, an explanation of food supplements, vitamins and minerals, information on which brands are specifically recommended and notes on the healing properties of food.

Foreword

As a busy physician I do not always have the time to discuss in detail aspects of nutrition relating to health for each individual patient except in those who come for preconceptual care. Therefore I am delighted that Martin Felt has developed a system of analysis of food values including that of trace elements so that we can all understand day to day nutrition.

As we cook for ourselves and our families we automatically include those foods that each individual likes best. There are some children who for instance hate eggs or broccoli and others who especially favour ketchup and chocolate ice cream and who feel deprived if these items are not on offer daily. Those food habits we choose as children and teenagers stay with us as adults and some of them are very wise indeed. Our brains sometimes tend to give us appetites for those nutrients we need like jungle animals at a salt lick but sometimes our appetites stray and we become self indulgent alcoholics or chocoholics and then we need the Felt Formula of understanding and retraining our appetites. When some special stress comes such as heart disease or cancer then again we need to relearn to pay attention to really appropriate and nutritious food for ourselves.

Those of you who can diligently study Martin Felt's book will learn in its pages the basis of a wise approach to human eating. Food has two main functions for most mammals: the celebration of eating with friends and family, the means of staying alive. It is essential to life, as are clean air and clean water. Those of us who are interested in caring for our own body and our own health will also be interested in practising good husbandry for our planet.

As a physician and a wife and mother I greatly appreciate Martin Felt's diligent and serious approach to nutrition for the third millennium. I wish this book and all who read it happy eating.

Norma Williams MD (USA) MBBS LRCP MRCS (UK)
Medical Director American Women's Health Center, London, UK
author – *A New Guide to Women's Health*
> 1984 McDonald (UK)
> 1985 Chartwell (USA)

> *How to keep a Mood Menstrual Diary*
> AWHC 1990

Social Inventions prize for Medicine 1990

Introduction

Over the last 20 years I have been exploring a variety of theories concerning nutrition ranging from the dietician's simple eating plan through the modern science of nutrition to the complexities of Japanese, Chinese and East Indian traditional systems. Before coming to Britain I spent a decade working in clinical medical nutrition and dietary research, eventually setting up the Alternative Center for Health Education in Philadelphia, Pennsylvania. My discoveries have proved to me that many of our physical and mental ailments can clearly be attributed to the foods we do or do not eat.

Having treated literally thousands of clients, each with their own symptom and disease patterns, my observations eventually gave me the incentive to create a system of balanced nutrition to counteract the pressures of a changing planet, a toxic environment and the stressful twentieth century lifestyle which are factors too long ignored as major influences on bodily health.

Refining my system of balanced nutrition has strengthened my belief that chemical patterns reflecting our physical and emotional life history are deeply encoded in each of our individual cell structures. These chemical patterns must be taken into account in our choice of foods if an optimal state of good health, physical and mental well-being is to be attained.

It is my intention with this book to introduce the idea of treating food as a friend. Within my practice time and time again my clients have expressed to me their confusion, anxieties and frustrations concerning food. They believe that if they can only make themselves walk a road of deprivation and sacrifice they will be rewarded with the weight reduction, boundless energy and stable health they most desire. However, I firmly believe that where there is fear and guilt in relation to eating then good food can turn to poison.

THE FELT FORMULA gives you the chance to understand

your body. By interpreting your symptoms you can discover your particular nutritional needs and requirements. The eating programmes are easy to follow and you can have as much as you like, safe in the knowledge that each product you consume offers you the chemical balance you need to achieve both highest levels of fitness and energy and your desired body weight.

The magic is in the food!

Martin Felt
London

Part One

CHAPTER 1

The Global View

'Those who rebel against the basic rules of the universe sever their own roots and ruin their true selves.'
Yellow Emperor's Classic of Internal Medicine

As time passes, the world changes. Human beings use raw materials from the Earth to manufacture goods, and produce the power that supports this manufacturing industry. The early beginnings of manufacturing in the West in the eighteenth and nineteenth centuries were small, but witnessed the expansion of towns into cities as people left the land to earn the rich rewards that factories had to offer. Agriculture, too, became mechanised, and farming populations dwindled.

Industrial developments of the last 50 years have been particularly fast moving. From small beginnings, the advance of technology has snowballed, and the speed of change has accelerated, so that the world we now inhabit is characterised by non-stop commerce, hi-tech manufacture, and a struggle to produce power by any means necessary to 'feed the machine'. We have become extremely clever at using technology by tapping into the processes of the natural world. But the waste products from this technology are fed back into the atmosphere, and into the soil. The conditions on the surface of our planet have changed, affecting the air that we breathe, the food that we eat, the noise levels that we experience. As a result, human beings have also changed. We live in stressful environments, and take in polluted food and air. As our bodies try to adjust to these rapidly changing circumstances, we produce symptoms that indicate that a struggle is going on inside. This chapter gives the background to the environmental changes that have given rise to our current situation. It explains the need to think about how individuals can remedy the situation, protect themselves from illness and regain excellent health.

THE FELT FORMULA is built upon the basis that there must be in nature, for each person adversely affected by stress and pollution, a solution for health. The most important thing to learn is how to combat the effects; what foods to eat in order for the body to maintain the balance of health.

In the last 50 years, gadgets such as televisions, radios and microwave ovens, that harness the energy of the electromagnetic spectrum, have been introduced into our homes. Little is said about the increased presence of the waves of energy that now surround us, inside and outside the house. Microwaves used in telecommunications rely on massive towers to relay the signals around the globe. Some of them are bounced off satellites in outer space. Simply, microwaves form a particular band of electromagnetic energy. This is a frequency that you cannot feel, taste, touch or smell; it is invisible to the naked eye. Being exposed to this band of energy appears to speed up the ageing process. Recent talk about mobile phones has suggested that the microwave energy that they use may be carcinogenic. A study of city workers showed that they were suffering from unusual stress syndromes, featuring noticeable mood swings, blood sugar problems, including an unusually high incidence of diabetes, and depression. Even the incidence of cancer was significantly higher than normal. It is known that if the seals on a microwave oven are inefficient, leakage is possible, and this is very dangerous. This is because the body processes and mechanisms of the cardiovascular system are regulated on bands of electromagnetic energy. The effect of microwave poisoning is to accelerate the release of highly charged 'positive' ions within the body. Positively charged particles, in simple terms, alter the chemical balance within the body. The body then needs to return to a resting point, or regain its equilibrium. Once it is opposed by some force or energy, a chemical push–pull effect is established and this carries on until balance is regained.

Without the sun, there would be no life on this planet. Ultimately, all the energy on this planet comes from the sun. The sun's activity – its combustion of hydrogen and other gases – initiates all life energy and is replicated in virtually all scientific technology. Our glands and organs, systems and cells themselves all transmit electrical energy. The increase in background electromagnetic radiation influences and transforms our cellular activity.

The constant discharge of nuclear energy and increased exposure to electromagnetic radiation is affecting our health, presenting challenges to our bodies that we have never experienced before. Excessive levels of electromagnetic energy overwhelm our bodies and on a planetary scale overload the natural balance of the air, soil and water. The main effect is to positively charge atoms, molecules and cells, creating extremely acid conditions. All diseases thrive in extreme acidity. All digestive upsets, for example, are due to over-acidity and the inability of the body to break down food.

OUR CONNECTION WITH THE ELEMENTS

The impact of the increasing quantities of electromagnetic radiation from our technological gadgetry is only part of the picture. Industrial pollution presents another source of change. This comes from industrial waste being pumped into the air. Much of what is contaminating our air is toxic compounds made up of heavy metals. These are dangerous natural elements that have been compounded in industrial solvents, which have been used in the manufacture of many products. Heavy metals are micro-nutrients that can be found in the human body as well as other life forms. Their role is to balance particular chemical processes. Excessive amounts of these powerful and toxic elements can promote strange and weird symptoms and can lead to disease.

Cadmium, for example, is a well known toxic element. The name cadmium comes from a Greek word Kademeia. Cadmium is used industrially in the photographic processing of negatives and film as well as being a prime ingredient in the preparation of many different paints and colour pigmentation. Furthermore, it is a primary ingredient in the electroplating of various steel and sheet metal used in cars: an anti-corrosive agent. Many of the processes of bridge building and welding involve the use of acetylene torches that give off cadmium. The best known source of cadmium is from the exhaust of both leaded and unleaded petrol. The levels of cadmium released into the atmosphere from modern industrial waste are highly toxic.

Cadmium exists naturally in the body in very minute amounts. It has a working relationship with zinc; zinc can help break down excess cadmium in the body. Cadmium tends to gravitate to particular tissues inside the body, especially the brain. Excess cadmium can be measured in the blood and therefore can be tested and analysed through a blood test. There is strong evidence that cadmium contamination is found in the air, water and soil, as well as in food. The most common disturbances from cadmium poisoning are in the brain, muscle and central nervous system, and symptoms may include mental disturbances, muscular atrophy, energy problems, sleep disorders and thyroid problems. This is just one of many 'heavy metals' that are finding their way into our lives with the potential to upset their balance. Nature responds by changing, or mutating, as a way of restoring balance.

Strontium, or strontium-90, another heavy metal, was discovered in the last part of the eighteenth century, during experimentation with calcium, for which it shares a great affinity. As a catalyst for radioactive substances such as uranium and plutonium, the effect of strontium on the body is deadly! Strontium destroys many of the important life-enhancing minerals: calcium, magnesium, phosphorous, selenium and sulphur. All these minerals are important to our bodies because they keep our bones and muscles – the solid, dense parts of us – strong and healthy. They are also essential for the regulation of the digestive process and the energy production from glucose.

Strontium poisoning produces cancer. Strontium is a basic waste material of many kinds of nuclear generating installations. It deposits itself in bone marrow, because of its atomical chemical change which makes it seek out oxygen. Strontium devours the oxygen from all the red cells in the body.

On 26 April 1986, an enormous radioactive explosion blew off the roof of part of the nuclear power station at Chernobyl in the former Soviet Union. One of the fundamental treatments that was used to 'neutralise' this chemical catastrophe (which included the release of strontium) was to pour millions of tonnes of calcium, magnesium and boron over the fire, to reduce the contaminating effects of strontium-90. In the Chernobyl incident the fallout was most dangerous to the inhabitants within 50 square miles initially, but then in nearby Sweden the results were and still are catastrophic in terms of the damage done to the cycles of nature. The fallout effect of Chernobyl was experienced in Britain in Humberside, Northumberland and Wales where sheep and cattle were badly contaminated for months and years afterwards. Strontium was and is still detectable in both cow's milk and mother's milk. It is also detectable in soil, and water supplies. Calcium and magnesium in particular forms can act as antidotes to this powerful element, reducing the risks of leukaemia (cancer of the blood), bone cancers and all types of degenerative bone disease. I am convinced that the increase of degenerative bone disorders is due in part to the contamination levels of strontium-90 in our food chain and the atmosphere in general. THE FELT FORMULA provides guidelines to help us adapt and protect ourselves from the threat that these poisons pose.

PCBs (electrical insulators), carbon monoxide, pesticides, herbicides, nitrates and chemical fertilisers together contribute 5 times more harmful organic waste to water pollution than do people. This list of dangerous substances finding their way into our modern food chain goes on and on, and should include the harmful additives and chemicals that are added to processed foods.

All these forms of energy are re-programming our natural body chemistry, in our own life time, and are passed down in our genetic code to the next generation. These changes alter our internal balance, cause premature ageing, and produce disease and the degeneration of healthy tissue. Energy problems and mental and emotional symptoms are just some of the early warning signs of how the body is being affected. Our future well-being depends on how we cope with these subtle energies. They will not go away. We must adapt. And we can.

THE FELT FORMULA is based on the ways and means by which we can adapt the physical and emotional body in order to act as an antidote to the harmful effects of our environment. None of the popular diets of the last few decades, such as the vegetarian diet, raw foods diet, fruit diet or macrobiotic diet, recognise the fact that the laws and principles of disease have so drastically changed in the last 50 years. As a result many of them are not only obsolete but potentially dangerous in that they may open the individual's body, mind and spirit to absorbing like a sponge the heavy metal waste deep within the cell tissue.

CONNECTIONS WITH NATURE
Thousands of years before modern material sciences existed, sage individuals observed, studied and collected data, and compiled them in the forms of stories that explained the processes taking place in the life-cycles of nature. For such a long time in the age of technology many of us have failed to realise our interrelationship with nature. All life is made up of cycles and patterns. Cycles in nature regulate the seasons, how and when we can grow food, when the tides rise and fall, clear and cloudy weather conditions, and the range of barometric pressures. Very few of us growing up in cities have ever learned how nature works, nor have we quietly gazed at its changes through the year. We are not conscious of the principle of Life Energy, nor of the physical body as part of nature in all her majesty.

The origins of medicine, however, were linked to the worship of nature and religious practice. Civilisation's first scientists were the shamans, witch-doctors and witches, who interpreted the meaning behind the rain, storms and other harsh weather conditions. They enjoyed privileges and secrets that the rest of the group, clan or community just simply didn't know. The early doctors worshipped and communed with stones, and particular land masses, plants and trees, animals, elements (earth, air, water and fire) and heavenly bodies. They hoped that, through their various divinations, chance would look favourably on them. They watched and studied the inexplicable and inescapable reality of birth and death, and they believed (as many still do today) that there was survival of an aspect of each person – the soul – after death. If that person was 'good' then they, in the after-life, could help the living; if they were bad their 'ghost-soul' would make mischief. They dreamed dreams, and the so-called experts interpreted future fortunes accordingly. These 'primitives' needed the assurances and good will of the 'doctors' and willingly paid the price of fear, superstition, dread, to ensure a positive outcome. Ancient peoples found meaning, support and comfort with an extremely optimistic outlook through the fates. Their worship of ancestral forces almost guaranteed their good conduct, whereas modern humanity has few assurances to live by. Today our practices seem to result in all types of human inequalities and social injustices, as well as political and economical exploitations and industrial and corporate piracy. What is there that gives meaning and purpose to human beings today? Do we know so much that there is nothing sacred to live by?

Without a knowledge of our connection with nature, it becomes extremely hard to arrive at real, personal 'beliefs'. Rather than understanding the natural laws that apply to all matter, our knowledge is gained through the advice of others. Rarely do we experience the world first-hand. We live by second-hand information.

Finally, now, we are becoming more aware of the interdependence between humans and the Earth. We are beginning to see all life as part of an ecosystem that is under threat of destruction.

Life was set up, patterned and coded by the forces that existed at the beginning of creation. Our bodies, and in fact, all life forms, carry this blueprint in the genetic code. For human beings to function properly and experience 'health' we must to a certain extent, honour this code by living in keeping with the way our bodies are designed to perform. When we do not, we get sick or disease begins. There is in the science of chemistry and biochemistry a chart called the Periodic Table. This table represents the material of our 'blueprint', the elements that make up our physical universe. The table shows the weight, measure, and construction of all the atoms and various chemical substances that make the physical universe. They are the very elements that scientists and alchemists in ancient times used for their creations. When these elements are found in excess in the earth they pollute the air, water and soil and therefore exert a tremendous power on our own bodies. If we do not adapt to protect ourselves from contamination we are in danger of absorbing these substances into our cell structure and being poisoned by them. Instead we can use these same substances to help us heal ourselves.

The ingredients or building blocks – water, air, earth, fire, metal – are all phases in nature that come together to create life. When any one of these is upset or out of balance it affects the whole.

LOOKING AT BUILDING BLOCKS

I want to give an example of how modern science theory is connected with the mythology of the ancients. The element hydrogen is the 'founding' and basic element in common with all life forms. It can reveal the inseparable link between ancient and modern, East and West. This link shows a continuum in scientific, alchemical and hemetic traditions. Using the language of empirical science, hydrogen is the most basic of all elements and molecules throughout the universe. Our sun is made of explosive gases, largely consisting of hydrogen. There is no life, as we know it, without hydrogen. Water is united by hydrogen. Hydrogen regulates the balance of acidity and alkalinity in all life forms through the ebb and flow of water. Hydrogen was the 'first' substance that was created. It came into existence at the beginning of the beginnings. From hydrogen, all other elements in the physical universe came into existence. The word itself means 'birth', creation, beginning, origin. The descriptions of the beginnings of Life in a number of ancient traditions demonstrate how it is possible to unite all traditions through a 'web' of integration.

In the ancient Chinese oracle, the *I Ching*, we see the following description. The First Hexagram (a mathematically based structure for divination) states,

> The movement of heaven is full of power. One complete revolution of heaven makes a day . . . Here the effects of the light-giving power begin to manifest themselves.

This description reveals the sage wisdom that hydrogen, the 'light-giving power' was the 'invisible hand' before conception, before any thought, before the beginning, before the void. The guiding Life Force that causes and affects all.

Looking further to the mysticism of Judaism we see a similar description from *The Zohar: The Hidden Light.* God said, 'Let there be Light! And there was light.' (Genesis I,3) This is the Light that the Blessed Holy One created first.

In the Vedic tradition of ancient India we see a modern summary of these 'beginnings' of hydrogen, in the words of one of the greatest and most prolific writers of this century: Sri Auribindo. This is extracted from his archetypal poem, *Savitri*.

> Into a far-off nook of heaven there came a slow miraculous gesture's dim appeal. The persistent thrill of transfiguring

torches. Persuaded, the inert black quietude and beauty and wonder disturbed the fields of God.

Sometimes poetic verse unites the scientific with the sublime. What we can find in every tradition and mythology is a description and story of creation that matches our Western scientific traditions. In fact, Western materialistic thinkers have based many of their theories and discoveries on the ancients, yet now work to disconnect them from the origin of creation.

What we can see here is the seeds of being able to connect one system, myth, story and theory to another by finding a common thread. By so doing, we are able to arrive at an integration. There is not only great beauty, meaning and significance in this approach. From it emerges the structure for a plan of practical action for change that recognises the living nature of relationships between people, places and things.

The ancient Eastern and Western traditions hold keys for the challenges of our times. In the history of Western medicines are these dormant roots waiting to be rediscovered. They have been buried and hidden for some time. The need exists to go back to these roots in order to go forward, beyond the new orthodoxy, our allopathic medicine. Collectively, in the West we have suffered long enough from being cut off from our origins. The wholistic approach has been buried alive, as it were, in autocratic medicine.

In conclusion, we can find the seeds of our wellness in this intensely confused and changing world. I believe food can be a tremendous support and extremely important in this journey of Life. Its chemical make-up is vital for our emotional and physical protection and support. Each disease that manifests itself can respond to particular foods that restore balance.

CHAPTER 2

Your Health in the Balance

Health means being able to eat the right amounts of *all* foods.

Changes in the environment have made a difference to health and disease (see Chapter One). Because of this, we must re-evaluate what it means to be healthy and look at the challenge that each individual faces as external circumstances change. Humans today have come full circle from their primitive ancestors who were mystified by what they could not understand in their external conditions and circumstances. Today we are faced with having created so many changes that we cannot assimilate them. All of us suffer from moving too fast and not recovering from one day to the next.

The most common problems and the most persistent symptoms and complaints that I hear from people between the ages of 25 and 55 (and most of these are women) are: 'I don't have enough energy, I'm always tired, I'm so stressed, I can't stabilise my weight, I'm all fluidy, I have headaches, my skin, hair and nails are terrible and they won't grow, I've been losing my memory all of a sudden this last year, my digestion is a mess, I feel 6 months pregnant, I can't stop eating, I'm craving sugar like there's no tomorrow' and so on . . .

Creation produced Life Energy, designed, programmed and genetically engineered to respond to a set of constant conditions in the environment. All individuals are 'programmed' to cope with some change, including those conditions that give rise to illness or disease. Even so, every individual responds in a slightly different way. These responses establish the boundaries of normality, and set the limits for the very basis of life, sickness and health. While the events of life fall within these boundaries, human beings experience comfort. Human beings also constantly monitor and control their internal environment, and the body systems respond automatically to change, as long as it falls within the normal range. Extreme changes in the external environment create stress on the body. Stress is any force exerted over the body that creates imbalance within. The level of our reactions to changes seems to be programmed within each individual. The sensory mechanisms measure any 'extreme' violations that create excess pressure.

Symptoms have an accumulated dynamic and are an up-to-date 'print-out' of the condition of the body, mind and spirit in relationship to the whole environment. Stress, or conversely, lack of stimulation represents the forces in the environment that are being brought to bear against the body. This pressure alters the shape, size or form of cell structures, causing changes in body temperature, overwork, injury, malnutrition and so on. In Chinese medical philosophy 'Yin' represents lack of pressure, or stimulation, and in chemical terms creates alkalinity. The most useful way to think about it is as looseness – or space. Think of all the molecules in the cells being loosely packed. Its opposite, 'Yang', represents too much pressure, which has a chemical equivalent in acidity, and tightly packed molecules. ALL DISEASES CAN BE CATEGORISED ACCORDING TO THE VIOLATIONS OF THE LAWS OF COMFORTABLE PRESSURE AND SPACE. Too much stress creates excessive pressure; too little stimulation leads to excessive space. When these laws are violated in the human body, pain or sensations of discomfort can develop, indicating a lack of harmony in the body. To begin with these symptoms may be slight. However, if the pains or sensations carry on for too long, because of repetitions of stress, symptoms and diseases become counter-productive and life-diminishing. When the body remains in an alert–danger phase too long, the ability of the whole system to recover and return to a resting point is hampered. The desire to 'get away to the country or the sea' is the body's way of trying to relax, or produce more space. Physiologically this restores the acid–alkaline balance. At the molecular level, hydrogen-based molecules become less tightly compacted. The opposite of this becomes true if the body lacks stimulation for too long.

One of the most devastating effects of too much stress is the effect on the emotions. There is the tendency for the emotions to 'shut-off', and for the person to become unconscious, in the sense of being totally unaware of what is going on. The nervous system, overwhelmed by stress, does not want to remember, and in some cases blocks out the recorded experience entirely. It 'disconnects' in order to survive the environment. One way of disconnecting is through greater stimulation – by tuning in to personal stereos, for example – which effectively cuts the individual off from the uncontrollable stresses in the environment.

Without the ability to unburden emotional stress through the support of friends and family, or redress the balance of physical stress, the individual is almost like a 'lone-primitive'. Such individuals make their way through the jungle, blocking out the outside world with an armoury of lap-top computer, fax and portable telephone. They are unable to interact or communicate with other people around them, or perhaps just find it too difficult.

Now, if you consider all the changes in our environment in the last 50 years or so, it would be fair to say that they have drastically altered the 'game plan' that our bodies had evolved to play in. This I believe is keeping our body systems at a heightened level of alarm, or alert, which is overstimulating and creates the need for a new form of protection.

Under stress the body requires more energy and produces fat in response to the pressure (acidity) in order to insulate and protect the nervous system from being 'electrocuted' by excess pressure. More B vitamins will be required to increase the flow of electrical energy across the nerve (myelin sheath). Calcium and magnesium will be absorbed and utilised as more glucose is required because of the over-acid conditions. Adrenalin and other adrenal-related hormones are released, making the blood pressure and blood sugar levels rise. They also stimulate the liver and pancreas to release insulin, increase glucose supplies to muscles and release energy 'stores' (fat in the form of triglycerides). This mechanism is the 'fight or flight' response of the body. Fat could therefore be defined as a chemical expression of too much physical and emotional stress.

One of the biggest problems today that has resulted from prolonged stress, is addictive and out-of-control eating patterns. Many people rely on an intake of various 'junk foods' including chocolate, sugar and white flour, as well as excessive amounts of tea, coffee, tobacco and sugar-based soft drinks during the day for stimulation and energy. At night the same people consume excessive amounts of alcohol, television, cannabis, sleeping tablets, antacids and laxatives for sedation. Many people who suffer from over-eating or eat the wrong foods are, unbeknown to themselves, creating a minor or major nutritional deficiency. The pattern of food consumption and behavioural habits creates a picture of addiction. But what is addiction? An addiction is a physical and emotional relationship to a person, place, or thing (substance), where no amount is satisfying. The substance gives a false sense of enthusiasm or a temporary feeling of well-being. As long as you continue to take 'more', you are able to go on. If you stop, limit yourself, or reduce consumption, the problems begin. The body and mind go into shock. The repetition of taking 'too much' of anything, in any way, to such excess, requires an equal amount of abstinence in order to regain equilibrium, the neutral resting point.

There is also the tendency during addiction to deny any dependency. Every addiction hides a deeper more complex problem that is unsolved and unresolved. The addiction represents endless layers of suffering. The real problem is a hurt, or a pain. The addiction makes the underlying issue a 'mystery' beyond recognition or resolution and so perpetually avoids confronting the issue.

The opposite of addiction is an allergy or an allergic reaction. An allergy is the result of the body and the mind trying to push something away. The body is unsuccessful in thwarting the ill-effects of 'something' that offends it biochemically, at neutralising the 'invasion' of a substance that is 'too much' of something. Chemically it is unable to make an antigen or antibody. An antibody is a protein produced by the immune system via the white cells in reaction to being invaded by a foreign substance. A body in a healthy state forms this antibody–antigen complex. For example, hay fever is the body's reaction to an exaggerated amount of pollen, when it has reached the point where it is unable to cope. The reaction of the body is always to produce symptoms. Symptoms are the body's way of crying out for attention and help when any of its glands and organs are disturbed.

Many people have a condition where they are both addicted to something and allergic to it at the same time. The longer the time of the addiction, and the more of the substance consumed, the more likely it is that the body, when it reaches saturation level, will react antagonistically towards the very food to which it is addicted. This is usually a chronic condition and causes great discomfort physically and mentally. No condition shows the modern dilemma and plight of the individual suffering more than this syndrome of addiction–allergy! We seem to have lost our way. We seem to have lost the instinct that is present in all other creatures as to what they need to eat.

Much of our relationship to food is psychologically conditioned. The stress and sheer pace of everyday living means that we do not take time to listen to and learn about our bodies. The stress in everyday life wears everyone down to feel helpless and powerless.

Illness or disease doesn't just happen overnight. Disease or illness is an ongoing series of (numerous) violations within the body to the point where it can't cope. Our health depends on a complex set of interactions within the body, mind and spirit. Our bodies are changing in response to the changes all around us. This means we must make deep adjustments physically and emotionally in order to adapt ourselves. At least 40–60 per cent of the population living in our cities has numerous, endless and hard-to-decipher symptoms that are not classifiable by orthodox methods of naming and diagnosing disease. They are not optimally well and healthy. We must search for greater levels of wellness, not just label our illnesses and accept them.

The most important thing I have learned over my years of practising is how vital it is to recognise without any judgement what physiological condition the symptoms are reflecting, and what is happening at both the physiological and emotional levels to cause an individual to be out of balance and out of 'control'. I believe that illness is a reflection of environmental poisoning, as well as of the fact that we just don't understand the combined effects of the food that we consume on a daily basis.

PICTURES OF STRESS
The results of stresses on the body can be described for each of the 24 body systems. (For a fuller description, see Part Three.)

1. **The immune system** reacts and so the individual's protection and defence is weakened creating inflammation and infection.

2. **The cardiovascular system** – heart, veins, arteries and capillaries – can become congested and all forms of circulation problems begin.

3. **The colon, intestines etc.** and all the eliminative organs become 'toxic' – unable to get rid of wastes from the foods and the environment as quickly as they build up.

4. **The digestive system** and all the organs of digestion become 'clogged' and so the assimilation, absorption and utilisation of foods become hampered.

5. **The sinus, ears, nose and throat** become congested with either excessive moisture (wetness) and catarrh or exces-

sive dryness and cracking skin due to the pituitary's inability to regulate and 'master', or control the external/internal stresses.

6. The liver and gall bladder are unable to process the 'dirty', tired blood, preventing proteins and enzymes from building up and breaking down foods and separating them for waste. This causes premature ageing.

7. The lungs, bronchi and the entire respiratory system are unable to exchange oxygen and carbon dioxide properly. The breathing no longer oxygenates or refreshes live cell tissue, or gets rid of the carbon dioxide waste. Breathing is hampered and stifled, not fresh and easy.

8. The reproductive system and sex organs become devitalised and unable to release and feel sustaining sexual pleasures. The necessary powers to procreate are disturbed, causing impotency, frigidity or related sexual imbalances. For a woman, the reproductive system is disturbed, causing too much bleeding during menstruation, or too little blood flow. For men, problems with the prostate may develop.

9. The skeletal and muscular systems cannot stand up to stress and tension. Aches, pains, arthritis, rheumatism, gout and cramping are the signs that the body is losing the battle with the environment.

10. The thyroid gland is unable to metabolise both the foods that the body is ingesting and the toxic environmental waste that it is absorbing, thus inhibiting the action of the overall nutrient coordination and delivery systems.

11. The veins, arteries and capillaries become congested due to low-level radiation poisoning as well as inappropriate and devitalised processed foods (most especially refined carbohydrates). Undigested proteins and fats also congest the veins and

arteries, leading to headaches, migraines and an overall build-up
of calcium and other mineral deposits throughout the system.

12. The central nervous system via the brain becomes
disturbed, which affects the activity and rest cycles. The
individual wakes up tired in the mornings, and at night has too
much mental energy, which disrupts sleep patterns.

13. The energy system and adrenal glands are 'drained',
producing blood sugar problems, and the individual can no
longer cope with everyday stresses and living 'under the gun'.
The individual begins to lose the battle with stress.

14. The mind–body connection is disrupted and the ability
to work things out, to solve problems and to use the faculties of
mind and body to distinguish inner from outer go out of balance.
Headaches, pressure and weight troubles ensue.

15. The entire **sensory mechanism**, hearing, smell, touch,
taste and sight, may have absorbed such high levels of poisons
that it ceases functioning properly, setting the stage for all
degenerative diseases. There may be a tendency for this to turn
up on the skin surfaces all over the body. Cancer or degenerative disease becomes possible.

16. The kidneys, bladder, urethra, prostate can no
longer handle the high levels of acidity. Fluids are retained. The
body clogs up and is unable to filter out the fluid waste, which
remains in the tissues. Calcium congests the vital organs and
glands. The body is poisoned.

17/18. The endocrine system and male/female hormone
balance that helps regulate the body's recovery from stress is
no longer efficient; nor is the hormone synthesis necessary for
all areas of the body to communicate with the brain centres.
Excessive sweating, extremes of hot and cold, psychological

'highs' and 'lows' begin to disturb overall balance and equilibrium.

19. The excretory system and auto-immune response have reacted to excesses of waste, toxicity and acidity. The skin is working overtime to get rid of waste; this is probably the result of the intestines and lungs being congested. Skin complaints show on specific areas over the body, known as 'meridians', which are energy points of the body where the war is taking place from within.

20. Now there may be chronic and long-term **energy**, fatigue and lethargy problems. Foods are not being utilised properly affecting the function of the **pancreas**. There is a loss of stamina and there is a real reduction in the quality of the individual's energy. They may feel 'down', even depressed. There may also be cravings for the 'wrong' foods.

21. There is overall congestion throughout the body affecting the Ph and the **water balance**; so much so that the body temperature and thermostat setting is out of balance, making the individual feel too hot or too cold, never just right. Foods are not breaking down. The whole body may feel heavy, especially the arms and legs, where there may be feelings of paralysis. The **posterior pituitary** controls this mechanism.

22. There may be **parathyroid, bone, teeth or joint** troubles affecting the calcium balance; including arthritis and rheumatism. There are too many poisons in the lymphatic system and this makes calcium leach from all over.

23. The **spleen** and **auto-immune system** are reacting to the antagonism from overloads and excesses which could cause both chronic and acute allergies to food to develop. The spleen may be swollen from the inability to handle its overload, which includes 'dead' and unused white cells.

24. The **lymphatic system** breaks down. A sense of not being able to cope with so much stress means food and other substances are consumed to the extreme. An addiction may establish itself. Tobacco, alcohol, sugar, drugs (whether they are the over the counter, prescription or recreational variety), are being used to survive in a 'zombie-like' state.

The above information outlines the plausible scenario that can happen when you are losing the battle with the environment. The questionnaire in Part Two of this book will help you determine where you are individually so that you will know how to focus your efforts to get back into balance. Everyone has symptoms of one sort or another. The body is working towards an equilibrium; it is therefore in a constant state of flux. These symptoms can be used as a way of tuning in to the current condition of your body. There is no simple, 'cookbook', way of being healthy. Real health begins with the willingness to take stock of your symptoms and their patterns as they are now. The questionnaire in Part Two will greatly aid you in this respect.

Healthy patterns of eating are established from the time we are conceived until we are approximately 6 years old. From then on, the 'software' is programmed and the ability to change our tastes becomes more difficult. I believe that I have discovered a very important law about the body–mind connection in relationship to food. We choose our foods essentially for 1 of 2 reasons: either to suppress, repress or depress our 'pain and hurt' physically and emotionally (as is the case in addictive consumption of sugar, coffee or chocolate, for example), or to help move the body to rest, neutrality and balance. These choices may be conscious, but are more often unconscious or subconscious. Healthy eating either links us together positively with nature and the laws of creation, or negatively to addictions and allergies. Each time we put together a meal we should bring together all the elements in creation: fire, water, metal and air. In so doing we re-create creation through all the basic foods! Food presents the source of tremendous power to create well-being in the individual. I have to be careful, obviously, not to promote obsessional or compulsive behaviour. The challenge of our time is to choose the foods that maintain a balance within ourselves as the world goes 'mad'. It may even be the case that some of the foods normally thought of as 'toxic', such as coffee, alcohol and coloured and processed meats, can be used medicinally, to balance certain conditions in the body. Food can help by virtue of it being the 'fuel' we need. Just like petrol in cars, foods determine how our bodies run.

In the field of pre- and peri-natal psychology there are amazing discoveries being made, about the education of the unborn child, that have tremendous implications for diet and nutrition. Simply, as a foetus develops inside its mother's body, the food that the mother chooses influences the creation of the physical body as it is developing cell by cell, gland by gland, organ by organ. For example, if both parents of the offspring are obese, the risk of obesity is as high as 80 per cent. Not only that, but the thoughts, feelings, sensations, pains, pleasures, joys, ups and downs become imprinted on our cell structure as we take shape and form. To a degree we are being 'programmed' both physically and emotionally from a very early age.

This biochemical and bio-emotional imprinting, or encoding process, takes place through the medium of the physical elements that make up our physical (and emotional) body. The process is known as galvanoplasty. When we are in a positive state, feeling creative, joyful and happy, the brain secretes natural 'drugs' called endorphins. This is the body's own 'pharmacy', which creates peak experiences or 'highs'. In a pregnant woman these 'happy drugs' convey the mother's positive state of mind. This is communicated through the placenta to the growing foetus and these 'chemical memories' are encoded into the child's cell memory. The nourishment process subsequently reflects this deep cellular 'software packaging' or cell communication. Thus life's forces are working on all levels:

1. The child's body is entirely formed by the materials provided by the mother's organism. Its quality is conditioned by that of the elements provided.

2. The mother's emotions are transmitted to the foetus via hormonal and energy channels (metabolic pathways), influencing the developing psyche either positively or negatively. The mother's psychological environment therefore influences the intrinsic quality of the child's cells.

The implications for diet and nutrition are staggering. It may well help to explain some of the influences on our 'food programmes'. Some people feel 'possessed' by a force that makes them eat foods that they don't really want to eat. This may be determined by the cellular encoding or programming described above.

In this regard, each of us appears to have a food 'persona'. This means that under certain conditions we choose food to obey one of the many 'voices' from within. I hear this message from clients all the time, especially those suffering with any type of addictive eating pattern.

The following are some questions to contemplate about your earliest childhood memories with regard to food.

What kinds of food did you share with your mother while she was pregnant with you?
What foods did she crave when she was pregnant?
What was the taste or flavour?
Was your first experience with food, breast milk or bottle milk?
How did your family share food, and what kind of attitude did they have to eating?
Was there a great deal of pleasure or joy in eating, or did your family tend to eat in silence?

What foods did you eat and what foods did you enjoy when you first started to eat 'solid' foods?

Were you allowed to play with your food and get dirty, or did you have to be 'perfect'?

Were you allowed to take what you wanted?

Were you made to eat everything on the plate?

Do you remember when you began to be conscious of food?

What, if anything, changed about your eating habits during adolescence?

What was the family eating pattern when you were a teenager?

Were there any problems or idiosyncracies that you had with food as a teenager?

As an adult, have you tended to overeat or be overweight?

Have you experienced the weight loss/weight gain 'yo-yo'?

Do you crave or have an addiction to certain foods?

Do you use food as a crutch now?

Do you have food 'persona', a good voice and a bad voice that are struggling with each other for control all the time?

By allowing whatever may be present at the unconscious level to surface by asking these questions, and then listening for the answer, you will become more aware of the thoughts that shape your mind in regard to food. When you answer the questionnaire in Part Two you can look more closely at the second group that you arrive at (see p.62). You may recognise these past influences of food.

By following the advice in Part Three, you may find that your perception of yourself changes. You may find that the answers to the above questions change over time, as a greater sense of balance moves into your life.

CHAPTER 3

What is disease?

Western medicine tends to treat the 'effects' or symptoms of disease, which often suppresses the 'cause', making it more complicated to treat. Eastern medicine sees disease as a 'live' entity that must be comprehended and understood in its entirety. In so doing the disease can be treated and transformed.

Good health requires equilibrium in the body, so the body, mind and spirit are always working to maintain a balance. Stress, environmental pollution, or eating the wrong foods can produce extremes of pressure (acidity). If the body, mind and spirit lose the ability to return to a resting neutral point of balance, somewhere inside the body a part will begin to malfunction as a response to the imbalance. During that time, the body will manifest symptoms wherever it remains under stress. Symptoms are the 'voice' of the metabolic pathways, a biochemical cry for help. The only problem is, you have to know its language. The language of the body and its symptoms is the art of symptomology.

When you do not heed the warning signs or cannot understand what the symptoms mean, they usually get more complex. It is important, therefore, to understand the significance of symptoms, in order to avoid serious illness.

The language that symptoms speak is pains (excess pressure) and sensations (excess space). Pain and pressure create acidity and too much space creates alkalinity (see Chapter Two). In the language of the body a person might say 'It feels as if . . .' This is a sensation. Or I sometimes hear 'it's not rational or logical, but I feel like . . .' An accumulation of these various different 'markers' in the body promotes disease.

INDIVIDUAL DIFFERENCES

For all the similarity of symptom patterns, each individual has a particular and unique sequence. Even people with the same diagnosed 'general' problem will have symptom patterns that are specific to them as an individual. Intensity, variations, locations and descriptions will vary from person to person. Making an accurate inventory and measure of these symptoms is essential in order to find the correct diagnosis and response.

For centuries, shamans, alchemists and doctors, especially homeopaths, naturopaths and Oriental doctors, have sought 'short-hand' ways of calculating and representing the endless variations of symptoms produced by the body. All these approaches have 1 thing in common; that of recognising that the body has too much of something or too little. Essentially, all symptoms measure the changing flux of hydrogen (see Chapter One) and how this interacts with all the other elements in the body. Certain areas or 'zones' of the body tend to build up too much energy or 'charge' in a particular gland or organ. That is why symptoms are always classified in relationship to these different glands or organs in the body (see Part Three). All pains and sensations have intensity and therefore can be measured. Disease therefore can be measured by the pattern and severity of these symptoms through the different parts of the system.

In real 'crisis medicine', the technology of drugs, surgery and all manner of life-saving equipment is fantastic! However, there is not the same emphasis on preventing disease and keeping people optimally well. This is the purpose of the FELT FORMULA. The questionnaire in Part Two helps determine the specific areas in an individual's body that are symptomatic. From there, the advice in Part Three recommends foods and food supplements that can be used as antidotes to the problems.

Doctors are rarely able to distinguish or recognise the different patterns and symptoms that 2 individuals with the same condition can present. Many patients express a feeling of being treated as a mechanical object by their doctors. They feel that most doctors either cannot, or have no time to, look at the individual behind the symptoms. A doctor who has been trained to emphasise the mechanical nature of illness, tends to focus on what is wrong with you and defines a disease. This is then treated with instruments, drugs or surgery, to fix it or make it go away. A more wholistic approach focuses on the opportunities you have to improve your health and quality of life and looks for ways you and the practitioner can work together to attain this. Symptoms are seen as a reflection of disharmony in your body's inner processes rather than a separate entity or disease, and a period of illness can be seen as an opportunity for transformation.

The real importance of symptoms – however minor – is in their combination, and in the hierarchy of their importance for the particular individual. Together they build a unique picture of your personal health. Biochemically every man, woman and child is different and so each individual must be looked at in such a way as to discover this unique flow and pattern. This is much more meaningful and important than putting a 'label' on the disease. Disease is a 'live', dynamic and changing process. Disease is not an event to be named or 'boxed' and compartmentalised, it is an organic 'entity'. Through misunderstanding the nature of disease, many people today feel that they are victims of their own bodies; they feel they cannot control the sicknesses that descend on them.

The organs and glands in the body group themselves naturally into systems. The following is a general description of how disease can arise in each of these systems.

1. The circulatory system includes the heart, pericardium, veins, arteries and capillaries. This vital system's function is the transportation and delivery of nutrients, and the carrying away of parts of the waste materials. The pathway of veins and arteries allows the blood to flow back and forth, to and from the heart. The cells are bathed in recharging haemoglobin, which carries all the minerals to the cell site. Born, matured and grown in the marrow or the spleen, white and red cells migrate in a criss-cross fashion, making their way to serve their task of cell regeneration. The circulatory system has command over the entire body via the bloodstream.

Heart disease is a major cause of death in Britain and the United States. One of the reasons is that the entire vascular system is being subtly poisoned by environmental pollution, and by the foods we eat. These poisons form toxic substances in the bloodstream. When toxins in the form of calcium plaque deposit themselves inside the walls of the arteries and veins for example, heart disease begins. The heart, in tandem with the kidneys, 'discharges' waste materials in the form of urine. When the body is overrun by waste, fat builds up in surrounding areas; the result is heart disease that can lead to a heart attack.

2. The digestive system includes the mouth, stomach and duodenum. This system's main function is to provide vitamins and minerals to all the cells. The body constantly replaces what is used in metabolism – the daily work of the cells – as it grows and ages. When the wrong types of foods are consumed the digestion becomes hampered and energy in the form of carbohydrates (complex sugars) is not properly distributed throughout the body. Proteins and fats are not absorbed correctly either. The liver, stomach, pancreas, duodenum and small and large intestines all work together to aid the proper utilisation of foods and the separation of food from waste matter. Gas, belching, flatulence, heartburn, gastritis, growths and ulcers are created when the digestion becomes overrun by undigested matter. All the related organs may become diseased as well.

3. The endocrine system refers to all the glands and organs that release hormones on demand. These hormones pass directly into the bloodstream. The hypothalamus and pituitary play the roles of commander and chief; both receive and send

messages to the rest of the 'army' – planning, designing,
stimulating and relaying information in the form of their chemical
secretions, but also taking defensive and offensive actions while
under attack from the environment. Via the pituitary, hypothalamus, thyroid, parathyroid, thymus, adrenals, pancreas and
testes or ovaries, the endocrine system gathers and sends all
its reports and information. All the feelings that you experience,
originate from some part of the endocrine system. They depend
on whether your experience at this level is positive or negative,
and this is based on your body chemistry. The most important
job of the endocrine system is to help every zone of the body
recover and be restored to a biochemical equilibrium. Therefore, any and all disease involves the endocrine system to some
degree. How the mind and body cope, and how it feels, is the
direct result of the work of the endocrine system. Human
beings who live 'under the gun' run the risk of destroying their
in-built hormonal reserves. Too much stress gives the endocrine system a formidable task of recovery.

4. The energy system 'To work or not to work', that is the
energy system's question and dilemma. The capacity to work is
its domain. From solar, chemical, mechanical, light, heat and
electrical sources, the energy system derives energy and
supplies it to the body. Energy is made available through the
process of oxidation. Some is lost in the urine, some is lost as
the by-product of heat. What is not lost is used by the body at
work and at rest. The production of energy never ceases.
About 25 per cent of food is converted into energy. Through the
activity of digestion about 5 per cent is used, 26 per cent is
assimilated into the body for use by the metabolism. About 7
per cent is stored as fat and the remainder is waste. The major
trick of the energy system is balance: not too much and not too
little. Through the ageing process (including the force exerted
from the environment) the body can lose the ability to make,
use and continually re-make energy. Lack of energy reveals an
upset of the energy system. Left unresolved, the body will go

into an extreme sense of physical or emotional 'loss'. All diseases indicate an upset within the energy system.

5. The excretory system is responsible for the removal of waste material from the body via the kidneys, lungs, liver, intestines, lymph gland and skin. Getting rid of poisons is vital to the overall well-being of the body. When waste, in all its forms, is not eliminated properly, the body can become sick and disease is possible. The kidneys, bladder and colon provide the means for eliminating nitrogenous by-products in dissolved forms. The breakdown of food waste, along with other types of cell debris, are dissolved and excreted. The system has to cope with the 'inner' waste from the body as well as the 'outer' toxins in the environment. The result can be devastating! If waste builds up quicker than the body can get rid of it, then these substances start to putrefy, just like garbage. ALL DISEASES ORIGINATE TO SOME DEGREE FROM UPSET IN THIS SYSTEM. The accumulated waste can begin to find its way back into the 'sacred' bloodstream, and when this happens the body is in trouble! This condition of 'dirty' blood, loaded up with 'garbage' sets the stage for decay and degeneration, and hastens the ageing process, preventing cell recovery and restoration. Skin inflammation of any type indicates a 'battle' being fought over the territories of the excretory system.

6. The immune system resists invasion from outside or inside the body. This is a twofold response; the production and regulation of specific immunoglobulins (antibodies) at the beckoning of white cells which join forces with their antigen (a substance that helps to produce the antibodies) to neutralise 'attacking' proteins. If the anti-reaction is too strong, histamines are produced in large quantities, which produces an allergic reaction. In the normal immune response, the white cell simply destroys the invading organism. If this response system breaks down, white cells can go 'wild' in a hyper-defence of the organism. This is what happens in cases of leukaemia.

7. The muscular–skeletal system. The body depends on the solid yet flexible abilities of the bones and muscles to move through space. If disturbed, these 'push–pull' movements lose their fine tuning. This creates excess pressure, limiting the body's ability to travel comfortably. Bones and muscles record the shocks, traumas or injuries that are sustained through the history of the body. This can be seen in the size, shape and density of the muscle mass as well as in the bones. Strains, sprains and stiffness are the tell-tale indicators of the body's battle against the environment. Arthritis indicates that there is a danger of losing the battle; deformities can be the result of having given up the struggle with the environment.

8. The nervous system controls the actions and coordinated movement of the body. The brain, spinal cord and nerves make up an endless web of telephone-like wires throughout the body. Responsible for 22.5 per cent of the energy demanded by the body, the nervous system needs energy in the form of simple sugar to conduct its electrical charges and so remain healthy. The brain, through the nerves, relays and switches messages on and off, resulting in a massive configuration of electrical impulses that are laid down by the genetic blueprint or code. The system spends all its time recording and analysing any threat posed by the movements of persons, places and things in the environment. Any disturbance or disruption here 'distorts' the body's ability to stay in balance and harmony. This can happen as a result of the nervous system experiencing 'exaggerated' stress or pressures. Such an upset may cause shaking, twitching, tremors and cramps. Ultimately this can lead to strokes, which are, in effect 'burn-outs' of certain lines of communication, where the surface of groups of the nerves die.

9. The respiratory system regulates the consumption of oxygen and the elimination of carbon dioxide, processes which are essential to life. The 'breath' is the most vital; it marks the beginning of life outside the womb and the end: the alpha and the omega. There is no life without the breath, and no breath without life. If the stable rhythm of the in and out breath is disrupted, this alters the movement of energy in the orifices and cavities of the body. The ancients in India called this force 'prana'. The Chinese call it 'Chi'. Luke Skywalker in *Star Wars* called it 'The Force'. In the alchemical tradition it is called 'Spiritus' or 'Spirit'.

The need of the body for oxygen creates an equal and opposing force, carbon dioxide. We breathe in negatively charged air; the out breath is positively charged acid waste. Disturbances of the respiratory system are synonymous with infection, inflammation and invasion. The sniffles lead to a cold, which can weaken the lungs and bronchi, and may lead to bronchitis or asthma. In very advanced and degenerative forms (which may be viral or bacterially based) the respiratory system may be besieged by pneumonia, pleurisy, tuberculosis or emphysema. Every single type of upset in this system can be traced back to the fact that the air that we breathe is contaminated by acid waste, which acts upon the breath and the entire body. The act of breathing is the act of balance itself. Breathing provides for us and makes us 'abundant' in the sense that the breath supplies the correct quantity of oxygen to serve our needs, and sets in motion a series of chemical exchanges, all of which serve the body's requirements. A change in the breath that reduces air intake is the first sign of 'change' which can warn of disease. Any upset to breathing distorts the senses and the brain. By the very fact of breathing we are animated and have all our faculties of perception.

10. The reproductive system is one of the most powerful sources of 'experienced' energy. The reproductive system is designed to 'recharge' the whole body through a connection to another human, body, mind, spirit, in other words, another soul!

The sexual glands connect directly to the endocrine system via the hypothalamus and pituitary gland. The sexual system can override many warning signals in order to fulfil its function of procreation. The reproductive system has an amazing capacity to 'Go forward' with a force greater than itself. The power of attraction and repulsion is a very physical power, which can move people closer together, and then apart. The well-being of the 'self' is very much concerned with these abilities or disabilities.

The disabilities of this system are strongly related to overall emotional expression, or aliveness. There are many things that can suppress, depress, oppress, repress and compress the healthy expression of emotional feelings in relation to sexual acts or expressions of love. Although much has been written on the subject, a true understanding has yet to be born.

This system invokes 'powers' of nature and beyond. When sexual communication creates imbalance in the body, the effect on the immune system is stronger than at almost any other time. A person's physical and emotional vulnerability places sexual communication under threat. Unhealthy forms of aggression connected with sex give rise to problems in the entire body.

Our decade has been saturated with endless stimulation, images, stories, dramas, traumas, insults, injuries, all documenting upsets to this system, which, because of its stressfulness, creates 'sickness'. This system is particularly sensitive to events and information in all its forms.

Women and their reproductive systems are being attacked by the low level radiation poisons in the environment. There is no gentle way of saying this. When the reproductive system absorbs toxic metals into its soft, vulnerable tissue, inflammations and dysfunctions such as vaginitis, thrush, toxic-shock syndrome, amenorrhoea (absence of menstruation), dysmenorrhoea (painful menstruation), breast cancer, early menopause, PMS (premenstrual syndrome), PID (pelvic inflammatory disease), candida and endometriosis begin to emerge.

CHAPTER 4

Balance and Diet

Maintaining a balanced diet is a feat in itself; considering how tempted our society is towards addiction.

Nutritionally speaking, eating a balanced diet is very difficult for the majority of people to achieve. Why? One of the main reasons is that few of us realise how different foods affect us individually. Nor do we realise the effects of each food group on our specific glands and organs. In the same way as stress disconnects us from our surroundings because of our need to 'switch off', so our attitudes to eating and to food itself show this same disconnection. The modern tendency is to eat for convenience and speed; we eat on the run, standing up, or while reading the paper or watching television. This reveals a disconnection, a separateness from our food; and the more disconnected we are from our food, the more unconscious of it we become. This lack of consciousness is what leads to problems with food or imbalances in our food choices. Just the act of being aware, acknowledging that we are eating, is important. I have talked to many people who can eat a whole meal and not register what they have eaten. Often, this goes hand in hand with problems of obesity and addiction.

Every religion, ethnic group, and culture has very specific attitudes towards food, and particular food habits. These are regulated by written and oral tradition. They may also have certain 'taboos' about food. Our attitudes shape our feelings about food. For example, in Tokyo it is standard to eat soup, vegetables and rice for breakfast, whereas in London this combination would be a very unlikely one.

Eating traditions evolved for geographical and cultural

reasons. The climate is one of the most important. In Japan for example, a macrobiotic diet is commonplace. Many Western people in the 1970s and 1980s had an interest in macrobiotic food. It may have been 'fashionable' to eat this way. But to impose a way of eating by dismissing one's own tradition, may not only be unhealthy emotionally, but physically and biochemically as well. For example, in standard macrobiotic diets brown rice is the everyday staple grain. But what works in northern Japan does not necessarily apply to Britain, or elsewhere in the world. This is because the climate has a large part to play in the way we digest our food. Londoners, for example would become extremely constipated if they were to eat brown rice as their staple grain and may start to look rather 'yellow', a sign of liver congestion. The macrobiotic approach has to be adjusted to the particular need of the individual in the given circumstances. This is not what tends to happen. The individual follows a standardised macrobiotic diet and this is where some of the problems begin. ANY STYLE, PHILOSOPHY OR IMPORTED NOTION OF EATING MUST BE ADAPTED TO THE INDIVIDUAL CIRCUMSTANCES, IN ORDER TO HAVE AUTHENTIC AND LASTING RESULTS, AND TO BE SAFE! This is important at both a biochemical and an emotional level. As another example of how climate affects the way we digest our food, consider the typical Mediterranean diet, which includes tomatoes, aubergines and red peppers. These foods help the body cope with excessive temperatures and also prevent the rapid loss of vital salt fluids, and are thus beneficial in a dry, hot, sunny climate.

However, in cold, wet, damp climates, these foods weaken the circulatory and excretory systems. Excessive consumption can cause calcium build up in the joints and muscles, leading to rheumatism, gout and arthritis.

This is stated clearly in 1 of the ancient Chinese texts on dietary advice. Any changes to the diet must contain a modification to suit the individual, and must be easy for the person to stick to. Otherwise the stress, upheaval and psychological imbalance, will make them worse than they were before they started to change. We know that all change (especially of the diet) causes stress. Therefore the manner of the change must be tailored to the individual, who must feel 'happiness and joy' with the long-term results. Otherwise a sense of disappointment, and of failing oneself may follow. Good advice today for dieters!

How could we design our breakfast, lunch and dinner to begin to account for all our different physical–biochemical and mental–emotional needs and wants? To begin with, we will talk about the components, and choice of food throughout the day. What are healthy choices, for different meals? When you answer THE FELT FORMULA questionnaire in Part Two, your results will indicate how to choose the foods that are right for you.

I have based my practice, both professionally and personally, on my belief that food is the best medicine. Each disease process, individually expressed in 1 person, requires (from nature's garden) particular foods and combinations of foods to move towards a balance and redress the disharmony. The plan has to take into account the climatic and seasonal differences of any region. Levels of activity and energy demands must be calculated as well. If you are sedentary and 'sluggish' less food should be taken. If you are very active and 'quick or impulsive', smaller amounts, more often, may suit you.

The single most important attitude to cultivate for health and wellness is awareness of your individual needs. Self-deception and denial are lethal weapons against a healthy, balanced mind and spirit. In other words, whatever you eat, recognise and be willing to see yourself as you really are, not based on the future, but right now! Each meal is a new opportunity to begin to nourish yourself and to eat in a way that honours the type of person you are.

Secondly, and as important, give thanks for the food you eat. Food is a gift and a necessity, produced by nature and designed by creation. Giving thanks actively or just quietly acknowledges our creation. It acknowledges our inter-dependent relationship

with the garden of creation. All other life forms can be taken as
food for us. When we take what we need it is a good thing to say
some kind of 'thank you'. Looking at food in this way encourages you to choose the 'right' things naturally and not to eat
more than you need. People tend to overeat for 1 of 2 reasons.
Either because there is an imbalance, a possible deficiency of
either a vitamin or mineral, or a need for more energy as
supplied by protein, fats and carbohydrates, or because it
stimulates or sedates a function in the body that continues
unresolved, and which represents a problem. Most people eat
to continue their pattern imbalance, either because they have
not resolved the underlying reasons for it, or just because it has
become a habit.

In fact, such attitudes tend to promote an obsessional–
compulsive relationship to food, in which everything is good or
bad, black or white. The real question to ask oneself is 'What
am I choosing . . . what part of me is craving or needing this
food . . . for what reasons?' Being afraid of foods, or believing,
for example, that you are allergic to a food, is not healthy. A
healthy individual can eat everything, no matter what, in a
healthy balance. Beware following obsessive advice on health
foods, dairy products, special diets, and so on. The real
question to ask yourself is 'Why am I choosing this food?' All
food choices should respect your needs as an individual.

All food is healthy if you eat the right ones in the right
balance. There are no healthy or unhealthy foods. Even the
terrible junk foods, if you eat a small amount, where's the
problem? This ultra-healthy, high and mighty, American
imported notion, is unrealistic and untrue.

Many people today have decided from what they've read that
dairy products are bad. Butter, cheese and other milk products,
including yoghurt and cottage cheese, have been cut out,
sometimes because of catarrh trouble, sometimes to control the
intake of fat. In either case, the long-term abstinence from
these or any foods results in the body no longer being able to
digest them. Such exclusion diets are not recommended.

Yoghurt in particular, whether it contains acidophilus or bifidus bacteria or others, is excellent for promoting good digestion and a stable presence of intestinal bacteria. It may also be helpful treatment for bowel problems and some digestive disorders.

We need to adapt our diets to cope with the threat of poisons in the environment, especially atmospheric pollution, ultra-violet light, and a host of carcinogens that surround us. By starting with a basic diet that is balanced, we can adapt our food choices to the various changes around us based on temperature, season and climate, income and lifestyle. These changes should always be moderate.

BASIC GUIDELINES FOR A BALANCED DIET
There are basic guidelines to help you first avoid under-eating or over-eating. Fasting, raw food diets, fruit diets and un-individualised Oriental eating regimes, should be avoided. Learn to eat all foods in a moderate way. The main goal is to avoid addictive patterns of eating too much sugar, starch, proteins, breads, chocolate, coffee and so on. But do not feel that any of these is completely disallowed. Learn to take them, but in small amounts. Avoid packaged foods with preservatives. Limit your consumption of white flour, or products containing white sugar, such as biscuits, cakes, crackers, white pasta, white breads and white flour pastries. Decrease your consumption of saturated fats, especially in the form of red meat, pork, ham, luncheon meats, fried foods, cooked oil, cream, sour cream and cheese. Avoid table salt; use a minimum of pure crystal sea salt instead.

Breakfast
The first meal of the day should be based on carbohydrates. If the weather is very warm and sunny, fruit would be a good choice. If not, then a breakfast based on grain is more appropriate. This could be in the form of toast, or cereals such as muesli. Avoid white flour, white sugar, sugary drinks and juices that are not pure fruit juice. A fried or grilled breakfast of

eggs, bacon, sausage and chips, for example, should only be eaten once in 7 days.

Lunch

Lunch is the most important meal of the day, eaten in the middle of the 24-hour cycle, at the 'core' eating time. It is important to eat well to give you stamina for the remainder of the day. Unless you are following one of the diets suggested below, concentrate on proteins for lunch, as too much carbohydrate can make you sluggish.

The suggested lunches should both be accompanied by green salad. Leafy raw salad vegetables such as lettuce, rocket, radiccio, parsley, watercress or mustard and cress, contain high concentrations of enzymes which promote good digestion.

1. Sandwich made from whole grain bread and containing tuna, turkey, chicken, egg, prawns, feta, ricotta or cottage cheese, with salad as above. Avoid tomatoes, salad cream, mayonnaise.

2. Grilled fresh fish, chicken, lamb, with salad as above, or 3 steamed vegetables, chosen from carrots, green beans, peas, broccoli, mange touts, parsnips, chinese cabbage, courgettes.

For a lighter lunch eat green salad with steamed vegetables as above.

Dinner

Base your dinner on carbohydrate if you concentrated on protein at lunch, or vice versa. This promotes better digestion, since the metabolism slows down in the evening and during sleep. For the same reason, do not over-eat at dinner, but be sensitive to your body's needs.

Examples of carbohydrate-based dinner menus are pasta, jacket potato, risotto, millet, buckwheat or buckwheat noodles, with pesto or an olive oil and vegetable sauce. Accompany this with greens, and leafy salad such as rocket, radiccio, watercress etc, as recommended for lunch, to aid digestion. For bulk, add 2 or 3 cooked vegetables from the list given in the lunch menu.

Snacks

If you have to miss a meal or you feel hungry between meals, eat some yoghurt with a combination of nuts, seeds and fruits, such as almonds, sunflower seeds, pumpkin seeds, raisins or sultanas. Crispbreads, oatcakes and rice cakes are also healthy snack-type foods.

Eat fruit in preference to chocolate or fizzy drinks, but no more than 3 pieces per day, as too much fruit can cause blood sugar problems. Dried fruit is particularly high in sugar. Fruit is best eaten in warm, dry, sunny weather; if it is wet, damp or cold, raw fruits will make the body cold. If there is any bloating in the stomach, headaches or skin problems, reduce your fruit intake to only 2 pieces every few days.

The 2 basic balanced diets that follow are, first, based on protein for weight reduction and, second, based on carbohydrate for building energy. They can be used either on their own, to pursue 1 goal, or they can be alternated. If you have major physical energy needs you may need to focus on the energy building diet, which includes more carbohydrates. If you have 'mental' problems or emotional instability, you need regular portions of protein. If both exist then balance the 2 on alternate days. First a 2:1 ratio of protein to carbohydrate and then the other way round.

Each meal should have the following constituents.

Protein base

25%	fish, chicken, lamb/beef
25%	cooked vegetables
15%	raw green salad
10%	soup – sea vegetable
5–10%	dessert
0–5%	water
5–10%	wine (optional) red

Carbohydrate base

25%	pasta, rice, millet, tabouleh, risotto, jacket potato, portion of squash (tubers, gourds and pumpkin)
20–25%	cooked green vegetable
10–15%	raw greens
5–10%	dessert
0–5%	water
5–10%	wine (optional) white

OTHER IMPORTANT GROUND RULES

There is an overall tendency in our modern, hectic lifestyles, to eat 'on the run', or to 'graze' on a series of junk food snacks, rather than eating well-balanced meals of whole complete foods. These 'snacking' habits tend to make the body feel out of balance. For example, if you do not eat a proper lunch you are likely to have little energy later in the afternoon and into the evening, and your sleep may well be disturbed.

Generally, the simpler the food, the better. Over-cooked, over-processed, over-complicated foods are to be avoided. For example, eat only fresh fruits and vegetables and avoid tinned varieties, with the exception of tinned tomatoes which can be used in sauces. However, tinned simple proteins, such as tuna, salmon and sardines are both nutritious and convenient.

If it is not possible to base a meal on either carbohydrate or protein, as recommended in the lunch and dinner menus above, then try to eat either 50 per cent less of carbohydrate than protein, or 50 per cent less protein to carbohydrate in your meal to aid digestion.

If you cannot stick to your diet plan or the basic guidelines in some situation, or you find you have to skip a meal, do not worry. The key is always to eat the best that you can under the circumstances.

ANCIENT NUTRITION THEORY

THE FELT FORMULA derives from a combination of modern

nutritional science and ancient tradition. There is great wisdom in some of the laws and principles of food and disease of the ancients. Essentially, because the produce of the natural world provided the available medicines of their times, these sage men and women experimented, classified and organised all natural substances. Foods were given categories according to the type of 'energy' they offered. They recognised a corresponding likeness of a particular substance to some activity, function, colour, smell, taste, and to a gland, organ, fluid or matter from which the body is made. Even the foods in each category have a corresponding likeness. Both the Chinese and Indians used a simple computing device that described 5 elements, 5 phases or 5 cycles in nature. These referred to the way in which everything affected everything else. Each element or phase corresponds to a group of related organs and foods.

Indian philosophy had another version of the same story. This story came from their myth of creation laid down in what are known as the Vedanta and the Tantra writings. In simple terms, all things came from the primal force called Prana. This force, or fire, created 3 forms, or gunas; first Sattva, the gentle and mild, second, Rajas medium to strong, and third, Tamas, very strong, or concentrated. These 3 forces react together to produce harmony and neutrality. In terms of food, Sattva refers to very light, airy or watery substances such as simple fruits and vegetables. Rajas foods are grains, beans, vegetables, fruit and occasional meat. A Tamas-style diet contains a lot of cooked meat, and heavy oily foods.

The Rajas is the energy necessary to 'break things up and apart'. Translated this means taking the one and making into the many, the freeing of the energy from food. It is the force that sets energy into motion. By contrast, Sattva is the original urge, or 'hunger'. In terms of food, Sattva is the lightest, gentlest, and contains nothing too stimulating. This comes from the Vedic tradition, where it was recognised that the least stimulating, spicy, or complicated foods had the least stimulating effects on the body.

The body is the most highly organised physical matter that exists. It contains within itself and its biological systems all the cellular structures from every stage of evolutionary Life Energy. In 1 body, the human being contains creation and all its unfolding forms. For example, the human mid-brain areas have unusual similarities to other cell structures found in fish, amphibians, reptiles and other mammals. The liver is an evolutionary link with the reptiles, since it can regenerate itself if it is damaged.

The foods we eat should support the creation of Life Energy. The elements that make up the foods we eat need to nourish the body and to produce waste matter. The body chemistry creates a cycle of carbon and nitrogen production. Carbohydrates support the carbon side of this equation; fatty acids, fats and protein support the nitrogen side.

When the body moves too far to the carbon side of this cycle, over-alkalinity results, and when it moves too far to the nitrogen side, the outcome is over-acidity. The present condition of the environment is forcing the body more and more towards the nitrogen extreme. All disease and degeneration thrives in over-acid conditions. As the body's chemical energies are becoming more and more disrupted by the threat from the environment we must take precautions to adapt.

The chemical compositions of all foods give us a range of choices for every possible condition or disease that arises. This is a law of nature. In the Bible it says 'I have given you all the herb-bearing plants and seed; use them as your medicine'. Since the beginning of time, humans have been forced to explore the use of medicinal plants to treat disease. Foods have enormous medicinal powers if they are used in a carefully organised way, corresponding to the needs of each individual. This potential in food has never been fully investigated. The ancient doctors, such as Hippocrates, Galen, Avicenna, Paracelsus and the eighteenth century scientist, Swedenborg (to name just a few) observed the use of these substances closely. Without technology or laboratories as we know them, these scholarly geniuses used the science and laws of alchemy.

Modern day naturopaths and other food experts have written endlessly about food. In some cases they describe with great understanding the importance of food as the best medicine to heal the body's woes. However, few if any have talked much about how to cope with and adapt to the changing polluted environment. To a small degree, this is one of the basic principles that inspired macrobiotics. Macrobiotic translates as the 'art of living'. But it did not individualise its approach, and only offered a standardised diet that most should follow, with minor adjustments. However, a careful interpretation of these Oriental approaches, especially the Chinese, Japanese and East Indian, has given the modern Western medical community the opportunity to bring an integrated medical philosophy into the twenty-first century, combining advanced technology with all the ancient wisdom and insight into the way energy works inside the body. Making this integration is 1 of the essential purposes of THE FELT FORMULA.

ANCIENT PRACTICES

Many of the ancients recognised the similar appearances of certain plants, foods and other natural substances to particular body parts, smells and colours. They codified and categorised them accordingly. These links have created the foundations of all modern medicine, whether modern doctors realise it or not. Unfortunately, during the nineteenth and twentieth centuries ancient cosmology and medieval alchemy have been replaced by modern science. The deep relationship between humans, the planet and all living creatures was lost and replaced by an entirely mechanistic theory of creation. Darwin, the champion thinker of the nineteenth century, promoted his theory of the evolution of the species, supposing that this negated the story of creation. However, I believe that the laws of Darwin along with the creation myth describe together the link between spirit and matter.

The similarity of the structures of the human body to all cellular life since creation is a scientific fact, but there is a 'higher' wisdom that operates in the organisation of matter. Science has shown that our human bodies contain glands and organs that act as 'sub-brains' to support the body as a wholistic entity. One gland or organ secretes chemicals that adjust the chemical balance elsewhere in the body.

The way food is used in the body depends on the efficient release of the appropriate chemicals at the right moment. If the system is disturbed, problems begin to develop that can be described as too much energy being available, or too little. The role of each type of food in this process is described below. These foods are described in order of their level of complexity, from water, the simplest, to fats, the most complex. The more complex the source of Life Energy, the higher the life form that it supports. The order of the foods described below also reflects the balance of carbon-releasing to nitrogen-releasing foods. As you read about these foods, try to build up a picture of this relationship between complexity and higher forms. As the world changes, so the nature of our foods must change in order to continue to support human life.

THE ROLE OF EACH TYPE OF FOOD

Water   The medium that allows the movement of energy through the body. Its main purpose is to adjust the changing acidity and alkalinity of the entire body via the systems of digestion and elimination. Water can either inhibit energy formation by decreasing acidity or conversely can increase acidity, in which case more glucose is utilised in energy production. When extremes of acidity arise, energy is produced, but the greater the acidity, the greater is the production of fat. Fat blocks the action of water. When toxins build up in the waste material and are not eliminated properly, fluid is retained in the body and the energy cycles are disrupted. As a result, fats build up and are stored. Carbohydrates start fermenting in the gut, energy disappears, and the body is out of balance.

Sugar   The most important product of all metabolism in the body. It is made from carbon and hydrogen atoms that, together, synchronise the production of energy and supply the body with fuel. If disturbed it upsets the entire physical sensory experience of the body. It also changes feelings at the emotional level. Such imbalances of sugar (glucose) in the body can give rise to the risk of diabetes. When carbohydrates flood the system the body's acidity level rises. Under these conditions, calcium, magnesium and other alkalising minerals are pulled out of storage to reduce the risk of sugar burning too fast. When this reaches a dangerous peak, the body starts leaching minerals from every close storage point, even from bone, to 'put out the fire' that the acidity is causing. This is why plaque and calcium forms in the blood and deposits in the joints, in the long term producing arthritis, heart disease and cancer.

Carbohydrates   The body's metabolism breaks the bonds that join carbon, oxygen and hydrogen to release simpler versions of sugar. Carbohydrates are an energy source necessary for supporting red cell production. They are also essential to feed the brain. Carbohydrates may come in refined foods such as processed fats and sugars (with no fibre or vital micro-nutrients) or in complex form such as in whole grains, fruits and vegetables, which contain fibre and micro-nutrients. To adapt to stress, and maintain a biochemical and emotional balance, complex carbohydrates are a vital part of the diet. Refined carbohydrates produce a much faster sugar release than do complex carbohydrates, which break down more slowly and release their energy over a longer period. The fast sugar release pushes the body to use the sugars, and a blood sugar 'low' follows the initial 'high'. In fact, complex sources of

carbohydrates are much cheaper than the high cost of techni-
cally processed, refined sugars. If there are too few available
carbohydrates, the body's response is to call on its storage.
This can cause the breakdown of protein, including muscle mass
and muscle density.

Dehydration of vital body fluids can also occur. A fluctuating
blood sugar level can cause severe depression, schizophrenia
and a host of other mental problems, as well as a sub-clinical
hypoglycaemia. This can lead to poor concentration, as well as
body, mind and muscle fatigue and a host of disturbingly intense
physical–emotional imbalances.

Fruits, vegetables and grains contain good complex sources
of carbohydrates. Refined carbohydrates are almost always
devoid (unless enriched) of vital B complex vitamins, minerals
and fibre (cellulose). Carbohydrates represent the 'birth of
energy' side of the cycle, releasing carbon. Proteins and fats
(see below) represent the 'death and transformation' side of the
Life force cycle, releasing nitrogen.

Proteins   A large complex of amino acids, each made of large
molecules, support the structural continuation, maintenance
and repair required for hair, skin, muscle, hormone, enzyme,
and gland and organ function. Proteins are either animal-based
(meat and fish) or vegetable-based (for example, lentils, chick-
peas, seaweed). Most mammals require large amounts of
protein. The debate about how much protein is required is a
controversial one. However, these requirements are individual,
established by the whole chemical profile of a person, which is
the result of genetic predispositions, lifestyle and stress factors, protein output in relationship to protein intake, psychological dispositions, and past and present patterns of trauma.

The debate about whether to be vegetarian or omnivorous,
based on the moral issues, needs also to consider evaluating the
chemical needs of the individual. Many vegetarians risk not
being in balance physically, biochemically or emotionally! My
clinical experience, including the results from blood samples,

has shown that they generally do not know how to balance the foods, or cook the vegetable proteins so that they are digested. Because of this, they are likely to lack important nutrients. Having been strictly vegetarian for some 11 years, and having explored at length how to arrive at a balance, I can say most vegetarians are 'eating their ideas' about health, rather than eating healthy foods for balance. On the other hand, the excessive intake of animal proteins has been well-documented, and is said to cause heart disease and cancer. The answer as always is to find the individual balance. Many vegetarians are more concerned about their relationship to animals than they are to their fellow human beings. Many vegans, who eat neither meat, nor dairy products, and others who follow extreme vegetarian diets, including the macrobiotic diet, create problems for the liver and gall bladder function. To follow these diets successfully requires a deep understanding of Chinese, Japanese or Indian medicine, and ideally needs years of serious study. This is lacking even in most qualified nutritional counsellors I have come across. It is certainly not available in general literature.

As well as essential building materials for the body, protein is a provider of energy, including heat. Unused protein is stored as fat. There are 8 essential amino acids that are required by the body to make 'complete' protein, the primary units for human life. The word protein means 'first', it comes from the Greek name of a mythological god Proteus, who could change his shape and form at will. Protein is transformed to supply us with our fuel to live. For proper utilisation and synthesis of proteins, 8 essential amino acids must be present in the diet. A simple equation that has been used to determine an individual protein requirement is to take the weight in pounds, divide this in half and change the units to grams. For example, a person weighing 160lbs would typically require 80g of protein per day. Unsuspected deficiencies occur because of inadequacies in the diet, and as a result of pollution and other stresses. The environmental pollution increases the requirement of 'free-forms' of amino acids to support human life. However, as with all foods, individual needs must be precisely understood, measured and weighed up, based on physiological, psychological, emotional and environmental stress patterns. The questionnaire in Part Two will help you with this.

Fatty acids As a group, these are more complex than carbohydrates. Vast amounts of research are being carried out into fatty acids because they have an extraordinary ability to break down saturated fats, cholesterol and low density lipids, and so perhaps reduce the risk of heart disease. Unlike proteins they support all the major glands and organ tissue and may slow down the ageing process. They also work with enzymes, other co-enzymes, and vitamins to protect the body from pollution and the harmful effects of the environment. Their capacity to support the whole endocrine and energy systems has made the fatty acids a source of great interest. They also help give natural lustre and glow to skin and hair.

Once again, however, orthodox research is running the risk of losing the vision of the whole, and 'not seeing the wood for the trees'. Fatty acids have a chemical ability to change form as a result of changes in acidity or alkalinity. Orthodox research seems more concerned with defining the parts than seeing the sum of the parts in relation to the whole body, and the body's biochemistry. Fatty acids must be obtained from foods since they cannot be synthesised by the body from within. The acidity factor in environmental poisoning makes the role of fatty acids more vital. They seem to have a marvellous capacity to restore, revitalise and energise the whole hormonal balance and recovery from the day-to-day stresses. Some fatty acids are known to help many skin disorders (which I believe, may be due to low-level radiation poisoning), hormonal imbalances, migraines and other headaches. It needs to be said that no one substance alone has all the answers or is a panacea.

Fats Fatty acids and alcohol combine to make fat. These
are less soluble than fatty acids and, chemically are a more
complex group of substances. Because of their insolubility in
water, they create more of a barrier and biochemical opposi-
tion to all other nutrients. This gives them the greatest 'acid
potential'. Because of this they also have the greatest energy
potential when acted upon by other chemicals. The problem
with fat arises from the effect on it from a polluted environment, and the way that this interacts with our body chemistry. Fat can become synonymous with incomplete energy
cycles (see p. 151): cellulite, lumps, bulges and expanding
waistlines are all evidence of this. Fat prevents energy from
moving from 1 area of the body to another. It impedes
chemical energies, and stores itself in a localised area for
protection as a result of acidity build-up. Wherever you see
fat building up, there will also be undigested waste matter.
Fat is the physical answer to stress. Fat serves as insulation
against the stress in the outer environment. Fat barricades
the tissues that have come under attack from the accumulation of acid waste. It is the answer found within the genetic
code. As a rule the body derives 40 per cent of its energy
from fat.

There are many false health food notions about fat. The
biggest myth about fat is that butter is bad for you, and that
everyone should use vegetable margarines containing polyunsaturated fats. In fact, the body has a very hard time indeed
digesting these processed vegetable fats.

There are 2 main types of fats: saturated and unsaturated
(with the exception of monosaturated fat, most notably olive
oil). Butter falls into the saturated fat category, most
vegetable oils into the unsaturated category. A healthy
mixture of all these types of fat will provide the best balance
for the diet. Again, making hard and fast or extreme rules will
lead to problems. Many people today have become terrorised
and terrified by fat! In fact if fat levels are too low, the
individual will become 'electrocuted' by stress, physical and

mental (see p. 15). At the Institute for Orthomolecular Medicine it was found that many people suffering from mental illness had extremely low levels of fat as well as other nutrient deficiencies. Any diet programme that makes any food a thing to be frightened of weakens the body's ability to discover and maintain balance!

Part Two

The Questionnaire

Answer the following questions based on how you have been feeling during the last 2 weeks. Do not think for long about your answers, the most immediate response is usually the most truthful! Give each answer a score in the box provided as follows:

0   you never get this symptom
1   you get this condition once in a while
2   you get this symptom sometimes
3   you get this condition regularly
4   you get this symptom nearly every day
5   you get this symptom more than once a day

Group
Total

1 Do you get colds, congestion or sniffles? ☐

Do you have any diagnosed conditions for which ☐
you are receiving treatment?

Do you have pain anywhere in your body? ☐

Do you suffer from catarrh in the mornings? ☐

Do you have fever or feel hot to touch anywhere? ☐ ☐

2 Do you have pain in your heart or chest? ☐

Do you have arm cramps? ☐

Do you have leg cramps? ☐

Do you experience tightness throughout your ☐
arms, legs, chest or neck?

Does your heart beat irregularly (fast *or* slow)? ☐ ☐

3 Do you have constipation? ☐

Do you have diarrhoea? ☐

Do you have an irritable or gripey, gurgly or windy ☐
bowel?

Do you have days when you do not defecate? ☐

Do you have bad eating habits? ☐ ☐

4 Do you have difficulty digesting your foods? ☐

Do you have pain in your stomach? ☐

Do you crave sweets, sugary foods, cakes or ☐
biscuits?

Do you have gas rumbling and grumbling in your ☐
tummy?

Do you feel dissatisfied with what you are eating? ☐ ☐

5 Do you get congestion in ears, nose, throat or ☐
sinus?

Do you get excessive moisture in your sinus, ☐
throat or nose?

Do you wake up stiff or are you slow to 'get going' ☐
in the morning?

Do you wake up congested? ☐

Do you pick up all the colds that are about? ☐ ☐

6 Do you want to sleep during the day or after eating ☐
your meals?

Do you experience low energy in the morning and ☐
during the afternoon?

Do you feel impatient or short-fused? ☐

Do you look pale, sallow, anaemic or lack colour in ☐
your face?

Do you have either an enormous appetite or a lack ☐ ☐
of appetite?

7 Do you have congestion in your throat, chest or ☐
lungs?

Do you have any respiratory problems? ☐

Do you have congestion or catarrh in your chest? ☐

Do you suffer from breathlessness? ☐

Do you snore or yawn excessively? ☐ ☐

8 Women

Do you have any menopause symptoms? ☐

Do you have any problems with menstruation? ☐

Do you suffer from cramps, or PMT? ☐

Do you have any vaginal discharge? ☐

Do you have any fibroids, growths or lumps in ☐
your breasts?

Men

Do you have any impotency? ☐

Do you have any internal pain when passing ☐
water?

Do you lack stamina or have low energy? ☐

Do you have any soreness in the pubis or scrotum ☐
area?

Do you have night sweats? ☐ ☐

9 Do you have joint pains in your fingers, elbows, ☐
hips, knees or ankles?

Do you experience pain in your arms or legs? ☐

Do you get sore muscles? ☐

Do you suffer from muscle fatigue or muscle ☐
weakness?

Do you get tense and stiff, especially in the ☐ ☐
morning or evening?

10 Do you have trouble with your physical balance? ☐
Do you suffer with being clumsy, dropping or ☐
bumping into things?

Do you have short-term memory loss? ☐

Do you have panic attacks or intense emotional ☐
pain?

Do you get depressed? ☐ ☐

11 Do you have spider veins? ☐

Do you have blotchy, ruddy or reddened skin on ☐
the face or nose?

Do you have cold hands and cold feet, especially at ☐
night?

Do you feel chilly much of the time? ☐

Do you have inflamed veins or arteries in the ☐ ☐
arms, legs or bottom?

12 Do you have trouble sleeping? ☐

Do you experience any emotional trauma? ☐

Do you feel stressed? ☐

Do you feel confused, down, or have trouble ☐
making decisions?

Do you always feel that there's 'not enough time'? ☐ ☐

13 Do you get tired? ☐

Do you get distracted when working or studying? ☐

Do you feel low, and lack self-esteem? ☐

Do you feel drained by people around you? ☐

Do you feel nervous, ill-at-ease and in conflict? ☐ ☐

14 Do you suffer from head tension? ☐

Do you experience visual disturbances? ☐

Do you get ringing in your ears or any sense of ☐
physical imbalance in your head?

Do you suffer from mind/body fatigue? ☐

Do you feel a sense of aimlessness or hopeless- ☐ ☐
ness?

15 Do you react to light or noise pollution? ☐

Do you have any signs of ageing – cellulite, body ☐
weight, degeneration, etc?

Do you feel tired all the time? ☐

Do you want to sleep to excess? ☐

Do you have any skin disorders? ☐ ☐

16 Do you retain fluids and feel congested in your ☐
tummy?

Do you suffer from any yeast troubles? ☐

Do you suffer from any fungal infection? ☐

Do you have painful, puffy eyes in the morning? ☐

Do you overeat or feel sick? ☐ ☐

17/ Do you have ups and downs in your physical energy? ☐

18 Do you have swings in your mental or emotional ☐
state?

Do you have a dependency on sugar, coffee, tea, ☐
alcohol or tobacco?

Do you have upsetting dreams or disturbed sleep? ☐

Do you have too much mental energy in the ☐ ☐
evenings and lack physical energy during the day?

19 Do you suffer from acne or any facial skin prob- ☐
lem?

Do you get hives (urticaria), warts or swollen skin ☐
that might turn red?

Do you have trouble with your hair or scalp? ☐

Do you have eczema, psoriasis or skin patches? ☐

Do you have athlete's foot? ☐ ☐

20 Do you crave sugar and sweets? ☐

Do you lose energy in the afternoon between ☐
1 p.m. and 6 p.m.?

Do you miss any meals? ☐

Do you eat junk foods? ☐

Do you feel disorientated and not quite here? ☐ ☐

21 Do you have sweats in the night? ☐

Do you have swollen feet or hands? ☐

Do you have hormonal imbalance? ☐

Do you have trouble losing weight or fluid? ☐

Do you feel physically weak, nervous and tense? ☐ ☐

22 Do you have pain in the joints? ☐

Do you suffer from rheumatism or gout? ☐

Do you have any pain in the feet or fingers? ☐

Do you have swollen or bleeding gums? ☐

Do you have muscle trouble? ☐ ☐

23 Do you have low resistance to infections? ☐

Do you have trouble breathing? ☐

Do you have respiratory illness: asthma, bronchi- ☐
tis, emphysema?

Do you have any allergies? ☐

Do you take any drugs on prescription? ☐ ☐

24 Do you drink alcohol? ☐

Do you overeat? ☐

Do you smoke or take recreational drugs? ☐

Do you get upset and become over-emotional? ☐

Are you suffering from anorexia or bulimia? ☐ ☐

Stress Number ☐

Mean level norm (MLN) ☐

Group with highest total above MLN A ☐

Group with lowest total above MLN B ☐

HOW TO ASSESS YOUR RESULTS

First add the scores for each group and write them in the group total boxes. Then add the totals from all the 24 groups together to arrive at the grand total. This total is your Stress Number. Write this number in the space provided on the questionnaire.

Now divide your Stress Number by 24. Round off your answer to the nearest whole number. For example, if you have a Stress Number of 79, dividing this sum by 24 you arrive at 3.29. As this is nearer 3 than 4, simply round your number off to 3. If your Stress Number is 89, dividing by 24 gives you 3.7. Therefore your final number will be 4. This number is called your Mean Level Norm for your test (MLN). Write your MLN number in the space provided on the questionnaire.

Next look at your group totals to find the highest value above your MLN and write the number of this group in box A on the questionnaire. For example if you have a MLN of 4 and you see that your highest number out of the 24 groups is 16 points in Group 6, write 6 in box A. If 2 groups share the same score, write the **lower** of the 2 group numbers in box A.

Now look for your lowest group total that is higher than your MLN. If 2 groups share the same lowest score, write the **lower** of the 2 group numbers in box B on the questionnaire.

The number in box A gives the group of glands and organs where you have an 'acute' imbalance, i.e. due to excess acidity and pressure, in your gland/organ system. Your acute is your most 'present' out-of-balance area suffering from 'excess'.

The number in box B gives the group where you have a 'chronic' imbalance, i.e. due to excess alkalinity or space. Your 'chronic' is your most buried, least awake, past, 'lacking' condition of imbalance.

Now analyse your Stress Number (see below), before following the instructions in the introduction to Part Three to find the treatments for both your chronic and your acute imbalances.

STRESS NUMBER ANALYSIS

Your Stress Number shows how much pressure and acidity you are creating and allowing in your mind, body and spirit.

A Stress Number between 50 and 100 indicates normal, or moderate stress levels. Between 100 and 250 you have a high stress level, while a Stress Number of over 250 indicates that you are in danger of 'burn-out' if these levels of stress continue.

The treatments given in the numbered sections in Part Three for the gland/organ imbalances should be modified according to your stress level. Full instructions of how to do this are given in the introduction to Part Three.

Part Three

The Glands and Organs

The glands and organs are an expression of the potential in nature to create a perfectly adaptable instrument – the human body.

The glands and organs are the biochemical 'command centres' of the body. Their functions are to work together in a perfect state of harmony and balance, always restoring the equilibrium. As 'centres of Life Energy' the glands and organs communicate with each other and both receive information from, and feed information back to, the control centre of the brain. Thus they can be seen as operating and functioning as sub-brains.

The glands and organs that occur singly are more vital to sustaining life than those that occur in pairs. For example, you cannot live without a heart or a brain, but you can survive without 1 of the 2 kidneys.

Even the most healthy person always has a range of symptoms, however minor, which are surface indications of the body's complex physiological functions and help to build up a picture of how the genetic programme is responding to the environment. As you develop and your environment changes, your body responds and adapts.

Through completing the questionnaire for THE FELT FORMULA (on p. 55), you will discover your gland and organ imbalances. The numbered sections that follow give you more information on the significance of your individual symptom pattern and will guide you in self-help techniques.

HOW TO USE PART THREE
Once you have completed the questionnaire and computed your score (see p. 61) you will have identified the gland/organ

systems in which you have the most acute (present) imbalances and the most chronic (past) imbalances.

You should first focus on the area in which you have the chronic imbalance. Turn to the section in the following pages for this group. For example, if your number in box B is 10, turn to the section for group 10.

Follow the advice given for the gland/organ group, in which you have a chronic imbalance, for 2 weeks. Then focus on the group where you have an acute imbalance for 2 weeks. After these 4 weeks you need a rest period. Eat a healthy balanced diet (see Chapter Four), stop taking the homeopathic remedies and supplements, but continue with a good multivitamin supplement (see *Resources*). You should not use the questionnaire test more than every other month and you should always allow your body the vital rest period in between treatments.

Foods and supplements
The food advice in each section refers to the Five Phase food chart on p. 170. A further sub-section gives recommended supplements and their dosages, and also homeopathic remedies to help restore the body's balance. Homeopathic remedies are very effective in acute conditions as they help to reduce and release the 'excess' that is causing the acute problems. You should only use the homeopathic remedies for your chronic imbalance if your Stress Number (see p. 61) is less than 100.

The list of suggested supplements is extensive, but supplementation works at a subtle level to balance and support the complex physiological processes in the body. If you decide to restrict your supplementation, choose those items printed in **bold** type.

The dosages of supplements and homeopathic remedies required varies according to the amount of stress your body is creating and suffering. Consult the list below for guidance.

1. Stress Number 50–150, normal moderate stress levels (see p. 62). Focus your self-help on the foods suggested.

Reduce the dosage of the supplements listed by 50 per cent. Use the homeopathic remedies in the doses given.

2. Stress Number 150–250, high levels (see p. 62). Use the foods suggested, to promote detoxification. Take 75 per cent of the given dosages of supplements. Only take homeopathic remedies for your acute imbalance gland/organ group.

3. Stress Number over 250, very high stress level. A Stress Number over 250 reveals that you are in danger of 'burn-out' if you continue on this collision course with yourself and your environment. You need at least 1 week off your 'crazy, hectic schedule'. During this time and after, eat the following diet for energy and mental stress: the Protein Base for lunch, and the Carbohydrate Base for dinner (see p. 41). Choose your foods carefully from the Five Phase food chart (see p. 170), following the advice given in the section for your chronic imbalance. Take the supplements in the dosages given, but do not take the homeopathic remedies.

After 2 weeks, choose your foods for the energy and mental stress diet from the Phases recommended in the section for your acute imbalance gland/organ group. Take the supplements and the homeopathic remedies in the doses given.

The affirmations
The positive thought or affirmation at the end of each gland/ organ section can be used to feed and nourish the mind and the spirit, to help release, change and transform lifelong diminishing patterns.

Write out the affirmation 10–25 times daily on a sheet of paper. The act of writing encourages you to reach down into your subconscious and may bring a corresponding negative thought to your conscious mind. To change this negative response into a positive one, try writing the affirmations on the right-hand side of a page, and the negative thoughts on the left, opposite each other.

You can also write the affirmation on a piece of paper and stick it to your bathroom mirror, where you will see it when you first get up in the morning. During the day, call the affirmation to mind and think over it. Spend some time in quiet reflection on what it means to you.

GROUP 1

The Immune System
PHASE THREE

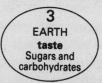

For guidance on how to use the information in this section see p. 65.

The immune system is the part of your body that defends you when any micro-organism, such as bacteria or a virus, attacks or invades you. When the first group of questions has the highest score in your test (box A) this means that there may be an acute infection or inflammation in your body, and your number in box B tells you where it is. When your second number (box B) gives you this group it means that the condition may be a chronic one. In either case, your immune system may not be working at its best and needs improvement.

The immune system is made up of the thymus, tonsils, appendix and lymph glands. The system constantly scans the body for any signs of invasion. One of the biggest threats to the immune system is the threat from the environment. Pollution and the toxic waste from car exhausts; industrial waste that reaches the air and water and settles into the soil; toxic heavy metals from all these sources challenge everybody's immune system. Inflammation anywhere in the body means that the body has perceived a threat and has responded to it by increasing the defensive mechanism. One of the first indications that the body has responded via the immune system is the flow of fluids in the form of mucus. This is called suppuration and is often accompanied by pain anywhere in the body.

By producing 'a wave' of sticky fluids, the body hopes to

capture any unwanted invaders and channel them into the lymphatic system. This system is a network of lymph glands and their joining vessels running alongside the veins and arteries throughout the body. But the lymphatic system does not have a pump like the heart to move the blood and keep it flowing. The lymphatics work with the movement of gravity. They can become sluggish and eventually congested when under challenge from the environment. But you can use aerobic exercise to stimulate movement within the system. There are also several simple, effective massage techniques to pump and drain the lymphatics through pressure applied to particular points on the surface of the body. The major draining point is located in the chest area just above the nipples. You can learn from books or a competent massage specialist how to do this for yourself.

The movement of lymph in the body keeps infection out of the bloodstream, as well as draining it from the blood, so protecting the whole organism.

Before the advent of antibiotics, peole all over the world died from 'fevers'. Fevers are the way the body tries to 'burn out' invaders (like fire) if increased mucus flow (suppuration) fails. The immune system has a strategy for every eventuality, very much in the style of the military commander fighting a battle. The strategy is like a battle plan, with a code that was engineered during the course of evolution and that is genetically built in. The thymus gland reacts to information from the body via the lymph with the hypothalamus as the commander-in-chief of the armed forces and the pituitary as the 5-star general.

Unless a condition is life-threatening, it is important to allow this system to use its natural defence strategies, rather than take antibiotics or similar drugs to get rid of infection. Children especially can suffer from the indiscriminate use of antibiotics. Their growing immune systems are weakened, and the bacteria present at the infection may become resistant to antibiotic treatment. New types of antibiotics have to be found to keep ahead of these antibiotic-resistant strains of bacteria. Anything which interferes with the immune response, or suppresses the defence mechanisms of this system, destroys, damages and limits the body's ability to defend itself at a future date.

Addictions of any kind weaken the immune system because the body uses so much energy trying to cope with being 'self-poisoned'. Addictions are an indication of a society where people no longer feel 'safe' and turn against themselves, or can no longer cope with the violence that is everywhere. Addiction is brought about when individuals feel overwhelmed by circumstances beyond their control. Control is the key. In order to cope, the individual takes some substance in order not to feel the pain any longer – in order to achieve a level of unconsciousness! Addiction has not existed before on the scale that we see today. Something in our world is terribly out of balance. When individuals feel so vulnerable, so unprotected, then addiction seems to be the last alternative – a survival of sorts, no matter what the self-sacrifice. The immune system, and particularly the thymus gland, has to cope the best way it knows how. This can mean putting 1 part of the body under pressure.

FOODS

Eating to nourish your immune system is not difficult; it is the most important 'medicine', and 1 you can really count on. Take care of yourself with the following foods: eat more Phase Three vegetables, both raw and cooked (see the Five Phase food chart, p. 170). Eat more Phase Two vegetables, raw and cooked. Phase Two supports Phase Three in the cycle of nourishment (see chart, p. 168). For at least a few days avoid the grains and beans of Phase Three and focus on eating small amounts of the grains and beans in Phase Two. Eat plenty of cooked and raw greens from both Phase Two and Phase Three. Eat very little fruit as this could speed up the detoxification and throw the 'forces' into a healing crisis. Many naturopaths and other health experts use fasts to help the body fight off infection or inflammations. This may have worked for minor ailments or conditions a hundred or two hundred years ago. THE FELT

FORMULA no longer uses these methods because of the extreme nature of the environmental toxins and pollution, which degrade the individual. Do not eat too much raw food. Look at the food plan percentages on the Five Phase food chart and use this as a reference. As you proceed, listen to your body, as you are really restoring your health.

Eat approximately 60g of sea vegetables every day or other day. This will give you quick and easy nourishment. As the seaweeds are a Phase Two food, they will assist the battle against inflammation or infection. Eat yoghurt every day at breakfast, to build up useful bacteria in the gut and bowel. Avoid all fried foods or oily, heavily cooked food. If you like, make some chicken stock and drink it like a soup. To do this boil some chicken in lots of water with green vegetables, carrots, parsnips, dill, garlic and a pinch of sea salt. Let it simmer for at least 45 minutes. Chicken soup is natural penicillin!

SUPPLEMENTS
Vitamin C is the best and cheapest support that you can give your body along with the food. The best type of vitamin C is an ascorbate form. This is mild, gentle and effective, more expensive than ascorbic acid, but much more effective at stimulating the thymus/immune system. For acute conditions of infection, take 500–1000mg 3 times daily after your breakfast, lunch and dinner. That may sound high but the ascorbate form enables you to take that quantity. If you have taken too much, you will get an upset tummy or diarrhoea. If this should happen, stop for 6 hours and take 2 tablespoons of yoghurt.

When Group 1 appears in your questionnaire analysis, inflammations or infections may be affecting your whole body. The condition has probably entrenched itself in 1 area of the body. When there is any known diagnosed degenerative disease there will almost certainly be accompanying inflammations or infection. Biochemic tissue salts can be a very useful and inexpensive way to help stimulate your own 'vital force'. Ferrous phosphate (iron phosphate) is excellent in the presence of inflammation or infection because it carries and stimulates the delivery of more oxygen to the cells. This is very important because the cells everywhere are having to fight off poisons, toxins, and waste building up and strangling the cells with 'free radicals', which are all the result of pollution and high concentrations of heavy metals in the environment. For acute problems take 2 tablets every 3 hours for 1 or 2 days and let them dissolve under the tongue. For chronic problems take 3 tablets upon rising and just before retiring for bed. They are very quick to help restore balance.

Zinc helps stimulate an increase of white cells to fight off infection. It also copes with inflammations once they have become established. Its power to work for the thymus and immune system is well-documented. Zinc helps Phase Three (stomach pancreas/Earth Element, see chart, p. 168) and increases the strength of the adrenal glands (energy system), which are usually low in activity during the time of infection or inflammation. Liquid zinc is very effective. Use a preparation that supplies 15mg per drop. Zinc helps form antibodies and also prevents certain types of anaemia that may be present with chronic infections due to lack of oxygen and a depressed blood sugar level. Taking a supplement of 50mg elemental zinc daily helps fight colds, fever, viruses and bacteria.

Vitamin A falls to very low levels during infections and inflammation. Vitamin A is a fat-soluble vitamin, but it is best to take the water-soluble preparations that are more easily digested. Beta carotene derived from sea and plankton vegetation is excellent. Take 10,000i.u. twice a day for acute conditions, or 25,000i.u. once daily for chronic conditions. If you use the mycillized form, available from select shops or dispensing centres (see *Resources*), 1 drop provides about 10,000i.u. and can be taken 3 times daily for acute and chronic problems.

In general, with infection or inflammation it is a good idea to take a B complex vitamin twice daily for acute, or 3 times daily for chronic conditions. Again the quality of the supplement is critical (see *Resources*). Average doses should be about

25–50mg B complex twice daily for acute conditions; for chronic conditions take 20–40mg 3 times daily. Additional B5 (pantothenic acid) can be taken with breakfast and with lunch. For acute problems take 550mg; for chronic problems take 1,100mg. Vitamin B5 stimulates the connection between the immune and energy systems, both vital to support the body as it fights off invasion and stimulates the defence by white cells.

Homeopathic remedies make an important part of treating any inflammation or infection. A particularly effective one is the **R1** inflammation drops made by a German company called Reckeweg (see *Resources*). If you are going to take any one of these suggested remedies it should be this one. For acute conditions take 5–10 drops every 1–2 hours. These drops can safely be taken by children.

The herbal product Echinacea is also effective for any immune problem. This comes in many forms: tablets, tinctures, capsules. Echinacea (also known in the American herbal tradition as Kansas Snake Root) stimulates the immune system to fight off all types of inflammation and infection. It is like a natural antibiotic but works without suppressing the body's own healing reaction. Take 10 drops in half a glass of water every 3–6 hours for acute problems and 15 drops 3 times daily for chronic problems. Bee Propolis works well with Echinacea; it has a synergistic effect. Bee Propolis is a resinous compound gathered by bees, mostly from poplar trees. The bees then mix it with a substance of their own and use it to reinforce the combs against invader predators from the hive. Taken internally in tincture form, Bee Propolis is extremely effective for sore throats, laryngitis, coughs, flu and fevers. Use Echinacea in combination with Bee Propolis when there is any condition affecting the immune system. Take 15 drops 3 times daily for 3 or 4 days. This helps with all types of colds and fever, and in general with any kind of localised infection.

Lastly, make sure that you take live yoghurt daily (containing acidophilus, bulgaricus or bifidus). This will help you fight off infection that lives inside the bowel walls. You can also take acidophilus in capsule form, 1–3 capsules between every meal.

Try using a positive thought for stimulating the immune system.

'I am perfectly protected and I can attain through my actions optimum balance.'

GROUP 2

The Heart and the Cardiovascular System

PHASE TWO

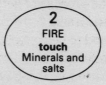

2
FIRE
touch
Minerals and
salts

For guidance on how to use the information in this section see p. 65.

When Group 2 appears in your questionnaire analysis this indicates that your heart and cardiovascular system are not in balance. The problem may be either acute (2 occurs in box A) or chronic (2 occurs in box B). The heart is the strongest, most durable muscle in your body. It is the 'general' of the circulatory system. More people in the West die from heart disease than anything else. Why are so many people dying from heart attacks and related heart disease? What can be done to prevent this? What is it that has changed so drastically in the ways that we are living that such a precious part of the human body is falling into such decay and disease?

Firstly, the heart as a pump sends fresh blood and oxygen through large arteries. Here is 1 major clue as to the problem. Everything about modern society, stress and environmental pollutions, is robbing vital oxygen from the atmosphere, and literally killing our hearts. The heart becomes blocked up with calcium and other unprocessed waste matter, and this gives rise to all kinds of heart disease. Varicose veins may be the first signal of these problems. Other symptoms are high blood pressure, phlebitis, arrhythmia (variation in heartbeat) and possibly a stroke in the form of a heart attack. It does not take a genius to realise that the concentrated heavy metals that circulate in the air, water and soil are likely to end up walled inside our vital corridors.

The heart is particularly vulnerable because it faces the daily delivery of all vital nutrients and substances from the digestion, entering and leaving through the bloodstream. The pumping action of the heart enables the body to transport nourishment to the cells and to begin the process of getting rid of waste. This is why in Oriental medical theory the heart, part of the Fire Element, was understood to be connected to the small intestine (see chart p. 168). Fires burn dense matter, Wood (food) and leave ashes (waste matter in the bowel). The Chinese also knew that both the tongue, and the quality and quantity of the sweat indicated the condition of the heart. Doctors today must begin to be trained in such accurate and ancient means of diagnosis. The early signs can be detected through human skill; they need not rely on expensive equipment that is not freely available.

The Chinese understood that if the heart was diseased or out of balance, there would also be a lack of joy, and a denial of love in the being, which could manifest as sadness or anger. When the heart is out of balance the body cannot be full of passion and power like the blazing sun; it becomes joyless, riddled with guilt and fear. It took 45 years to get the medical people to accept that diet had a link to heart disease! Still today the recommendations made by the British and American Heart Associations are so conservative that millions are dying unnecessarily.

Fats are the main culprit in the diet and the battle against heart disease. When all the fluids of the body become too acid (which may result from overeating in times of stress, see p. 16) then fat is the result. The danger here is to mistake which fats to use in the diet. Contrary to popular opinion, the soft, polyunsaturated margarines are more harmful than butter (see p. 51).

Drink 2 cups of hot water with a large squeeze of lemon or

lime juice immediately after rising. Take a brisk 40 minute walk early every morning on an empty stomach. Do not sleep more than 7–8 hours a night. Do not overwork. Reduce general stress and tension. Learn to meditate; take a course in Transcendental Meditation. Make a commitment to meditate for 20 minutes every day for a month, but have a goal to do it every day for 6 months! Take up some kind of creative outlet, such as painting, writing or drama. Give and receive at least 3 hugs every day, and ask loved-ones or family members to tell you how much they love and accept you for being the special and wonderful person that you are. If they do not want to do this then you can begin to understand why you may have heart disease; your emotional heart is 'hurting' as well. You may think this is silly but it is not. Look in the mirror every day first thing in the morning and last thing at night and tell yourself 4 or 5 different things you really love about yourself. If you cannot do this, again you can begin to understand why your heart is sick. Face up to this, because it will not go away, no matter how much you try to deny it or rationalise it away. Carry out these suggestions (no human being is perfect). Make a list of 100 things, persons or places that you feel guilty about. Guilt produces heart disease, whether medical doctors can prove it or not!

Realise that you have, up to this moment, probably been your own worst enemy and not loved or liked yourself very much. Consciously forgive yourself for this. You didn't know and you were not told any better. You learned to treat yourself this way and you also hurt yourself with food. This will help to reverse the self-destruct mechanism that can exist in all of us at times. We all experience unique and particular poisons both in the environment and in the food we eat, thereby creating our own disease patterns. You are only a victim if you want to be. Save yourself. Nobody else can be saved or helped by you until you help yourself. It takes guts to heal yourself, and ultimately, no doctor can do all the healing work. The power is within you. You should use it.

FOODS

When Group 2 shows up in your questionnaire analysis, in either box A or box B, then you MUST change your diet and do this in a moderate way. Referring to the Five Phase food chart (see p. 170), focus on increasing the Phase One vegetables, particularly the greens as they contain chlorophyl and enzymes that will begin to break down the fat and other waste matter that is clogging the system.

Enzymes are the key to rejuvenating a diseased heart and vascular system. Large amounts of enzymes from foods are needed to cleanse the body of fat and plaque.

Stop eating red meat for at least 3–6 months or until your weight returns to the right level for your height and frame. Reduce the amounts of foods that you eat at meal times by one quarter to one third. Refer to the diets given in Chapter Four (see p. 39), and rotate the 2 meal plans every other day, i.e. day 1 lunch–protein, dinner–carbohydrate; day 2, lunch–carbohydrate, dinner–protein. Never eat fruits and vegetables together at a meal. Do not drink fluids with lunch or dinner. Cut out additional salt on your foods. Spend 5–20 minutes relaxing before eating. Do not eat if you are feeling stressed or uptight, because food will not be digested properly. Instead have a small snack and wait until you are feeling better. You can have a glass of wine with dinner or a whisky before meal time. Eat small amounts of white meats. Do not take up any extreme diet because swings between weight loss and weight gain are very stressful for the circulatory system, including the heart. Eat protein for lunch if possible and carbohydrates for dinner. Eat protein or carbohydrates always with a green salad and vegetables. Avoid taking more than a total of 2 or 3 cups of tea or coffee daily. Do not eat white flour or white sugar. Cut out pork, ham and prepared luncheon meats. Avoid tomatoes, peppers, mushrooms, spinach, oranges, grapefruits, peanuts, cashews, pistachios and white potato. Have these only twice a week at most.

SUPPLEMENTS

There are many different types of heart condition and disorders of the circulatory/vascular system. The supplements listed are for general acute and chronic conditions. In all cases it is imperative to consult appropriate specialists for monitoring and treatment. Take a good **multimineral** (see *Resources*) every day.

Vitamin E is suitable for every heart problem. A recent study on dentists and nurses suffering from advanced heart disease found that vitamin E helped significantly to improve their conditions. It has cost millions of pounds in research to find out what has been known to some nutritional specialists (particularly the pioneer researcher Dr W. Shute) for nearly 50 years. Vitamin E is a fat-soluble vitamin and should be taken most effectively in 'dry' form as Succinate E. For acute early heart problems take 400i.u. daily. For advanced chronic conditions, use 600–1,000i.u. daily. There is also a water-soluble liquid vitamin E.

Coenzyme Q10 is another important supplement for the heart. It assists the heart muscle and heals the membrane surrounding the heart. Extensive research on this was carried out in the former Soviet Union. Acute dosage: 30mg twice daily. Chronic dosage: 60mg once daily.

Vitamin C is excellent for the heart because it has natural anti-inflammatory properties and helps integrate soft tissue, the 'glue' of the body. For acute angina or chest pain along with any medication such as nitroglycerine, take at least 1,000mg magnesium ascorbate 3 times daily. Any of the above supplements can be taken alongside all prescribed drugs. For chronic problems, take 2,000mg 2 or 3 times daily. If this dose is too high it may upset the bowel or your tummy. Reduce the dose by 1,000mg until it is settled. Always use magnesium ascorbate, not calcium ascorbate which may affect the heart.

Phosphatidyl choline is a concentrate of a B complex vitamin, choline, and is an important vitamin to help in the metabolism of fat. It comes in 1,200mg capsules and is the major active ingredient in Lecithin 1. Phosphatidyl choline also stimulates and activates the clearance of fat in the liver. Take 2 capsules 3 times daily in all related conditions.

Carnitine is an amino acid well-researched by several well known doctors. Dr Eric Bravermann of the Brain Bio-Center in Princeton, New Jersey, worked with Dr Carl Peiffer MD and wrote an important work on the use of amino acid therapy. I was a guinea pig for their trial. They suggest 500–1,000mg daily of L-Carnitine. This should be taken on an empty stomach. Carnitine strengthens the heart.

Niacin or nicotinic acid is vitamin B3. This dramatically improves circulation, and stimulates the fat barriers where incomplete energy is stored as fat. A dose of more than 100mg of niacin can cause flushing and tingling, itchy, prickly skin. Nicotinic acid does not have this problem and is just as effective. For acute conditions take 100mg every 4–6 hours. For chronic problems use 500mg 2 or 3 times daily.

Homeopathic remedies for the heart include Reckeweg R2. These drops are for cardiac arrhythmia (variations in the heartbeat), palpitations, myocardial constrictions and angina. In acute problems when there are frequent, severe irregularities, take 10 drops every half hour. For chronic problems, take 15 drops 3 times daily. Take Reckeweg R3 for myocardial weakness, degenerative muscular problems, infarctions. Acute conditions: 10–15 drops 4–6 times daily. Chronic conditions: 10–30 drops 3 times daily. In venous stasis, varicosity and inflamed veins, use R42. For cardiac conduction problems following degenerative heart disease, endocardities and tachycardia, use remedy R66. For acute problems, 10 drops every 15–30 minutes; for chronic problems, 10–15 drops 3 times daily.

For cardiac failure with circulatory disturbances after infectious diseases affecting the heart, vertigo or tendency to faint, use remedy R67. In acute shock take 5–10 drops every 15–30 minutes. For chronic use and after some recovery, 10–15 drops 3 times daily. For hypertension use remedy R79 in tonifying capsules with garlic and hawthorn berries. Take 1 capsule 3 times daily. For arteriosclerosis, use remedy R12. For acute problems, take 10–15 drops every 1–3 hours. For chronic problems take 10–15 drops 3 times daily.

Try using a positive thought to stimulate your heart.

'I am worthy of loving myself and I love my body, mind and spirit fully.'

GROUP 3

The Colon and the Elimination System

PHASE FOUR

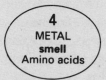

4
METAL
smell
Amino acids

For guidance on how to use the information in this section see p.
65.

The colon and bowel are responsible for the elimination of the solid, or 'heavy' waste material from the body. Working together with the kidneys, bladder and the skin, all cell waste is ejected via the excretory system. The colon is the 'work horse' of the system. The health of the colon determines the beginning and end of all disease. Present conditions in the environment make the job of the colon extremely difficult. Every substance in the air, water, soil and food finds its way into the colon. If the system does not work properly and efficiently, fats go rancid, proteins putrefy and carbohydrates ferment. All these changes set the stage for degenerative diseases. Chinese medicine acknowledges 'things going rotten' in the area of the large intestine by the smell of a person. This betrays how the colon is functioning. Also, problems with the skin are a sign that the body is unable to eliminate waste properly. In this situation the lungs try to eliminate what is not being eliminated by the colon, and this, in turn creates lung disturbances.

When the colon is out of balance, the whole organism is affected. The job of the colon is to get rid of the 'garbage', which is the positive charge; in other words, the most acid waste. If the colon does not work efficiently, poisonous waste starts finding its way back into the system. Individuals suffering from irritable bowel, constipation, diarrhoea, diverticulitis, *all* have problems 'letting go' or 'being released' from their waste. The problem can be at a physical, mental or emotional level. When an individual does not defecate properly and regularly every day, any disease can take root, depending on the individual, and particularly any hereditary weakness. Any skin disturbance is the tell-tale sign that the acid–alkaline balance and digestion, assimilation, utilisation and elimination of foods is out of balance. When these problems exist, the colon must be restored. When the colon can no longer detoxify the system, the individual experiences the inability to achieve this physical sense of harmony. Letting go physically is an important part of the vital force. It can be achieved both through the activity of the colon and the activity of the sexual system through orgasm. When the colon is blocked, the sexual system will also become blocked because they are so closely allied by their role in maintaining the vital force, creating new life and letting go of old life (waste matter). When the bowel does not work properly the individual tends to get irritable, negative, vindictive and hateful.

The whole action of the bowel and colon is a muscular undulation and movement through peristalsis. Waste matter is sent towards the last stop on a long trip, making an exit at the rectum. All along the way the bends and curves may create pockets where waste can get stuck. This is largely due to eating foods that contain insufficient fibre or devitalised nutrients. Much of the food we eat has been commercially processed in order to extend its shelf life (and profitability). White flour, white sugar, fizzy drinks with artificial sweetener, cakes, biscuits, sweets, hormone-ridden poultry and beef, are some of the most deadly examples. The environmental poisons add insult to injury, congesting and making this journey fraught with challenges and problems. When the colon becomes clogged up with toxic foods, and poisons from petrol exhaust, industrial waste and nuclear radiation, the stage is set for cancer of the colon, the second biggest cause of death in many Western countries today. This disease is the only possible justice when the colon remains poisoned. No wonder the colon is breaking down and unable to work properly.

FOODS

Problems with elimination affect the Metal element, Phase Four (see p. 168). To support the colon, increase the Phase Three and Four foods, referring to the Five Phase food chart on p. 170. Most especially increase the Phase Four vegetables, which provide roughage to detoxify the colon. Avoid Phase Four beans, nuts, seeds and dairy products. Increase Phase Two foods to help clear the colon and the entire bowel. Eat more grains from Phase Two and Phase Three: corn and millet (Phase Five grains such as buckwheat are neutral). This will have a rejuvenating effect on the colon. Increase the fibre in your diet dramatically if you are constipated. Wheat bran may irritate the intestines, so instead try some Linseed Gold, an organically grown linseed from Germany. This usually does the trick. When this does not work effectively, try a powder mix that is very mild with bulking and lubrication called Bio-blend (see *Resources*). Take these products before bedtime.

GPs often suggest simply eating more fibre. From my experience with thousands of people this will not give the desired results. You need to make a more radical adjustment to your diet, as outlined above. Reduce your dairy products, especially cheese if you are constipated or if you have diarrhoea. To protect the mucous membrane of the colon from excess acidity and the corresponding congestion, blockages, prolapses and general mucus build-up, avoid acidic foods: tomatoes, peppers, mushrooms, oranges, grapefruit, all nuts, coffee, tea, all pulses, rhubarb, cauliflower, cabbage, turnips, swedes, fried foods, mayonnaise, shellfish, vinegar, spinach, aubergines, all red meats and all smoked meats, and excess butter and cream.

Eat yoghurt daily. When the bowel is irritable and there is diarrhoea, avoid any raw foods other than a small green salad with watercress, parsley and cress. Do not eat too much bread or wheat as the yeast and wheat may combine to promote excess fermentation and this will continue to inflame the mucous membranes.

For breakfast eat porridge made from millet flakes or the whole seeds. Blend it with some yoghurt and a quarter of a ripe banana. If available, papaya or mango blended with yoghurt is very healing and soothing to the inflamed tissue and this could be alternated with the millet breakfast.

For lunch prepare boiled or poached white meat or fish with 2 or 3 soft vegetables: carrots, parsnips, green beans, green peas, courgettes or okra. Have the same for dinner until the condition improves. Alternatively, eat cooked white (or brown) basmati rice with vegetables. Add 1 or 2 teaspoons of natural live yoghurt to the vegetables, a teaspoon of olive oil and a squeeze of lemon juice. This replaces salt. One hour after the meal have 3 teaspoons of yoghurt in half a glass of water and a minute pinch of salt. Drink slowly. Take some Slippery Elm tea before retiring, which will coat and soothe the colon and stop the loose stool. If the condition persists you *must* consult your doctor.

SUPPLEMENTS

For constipation and related conditions, take a dried fruit product called Ortis cube (made by Ortis Company, see *Resources*). Once the work of your colon is more regular as a result of the diet and the treatment, discontinue the cube but continue the diet. Take a high potency multivitamin (see *Resources*). Take calcium and magnesium (chelated) in a 2:1 ratio 3 times daily. Take 1,000mg vitamin C daily, as either calcium or magnesium ascorbate. Take a digestive enzyme after lunch and dinner (see *Resources*,). Dandelion, Golden Seal, or Aloe Vera capsules can be taken for 1 week before bed. Two capsules daily will help regulate the bowels.

For diarrhoea and irritable bowel, take a low potency liquid B complex 3 times a day. In addition, take the Bio-Care Ligazyme product to help reintegrate the inflamed tissue membranes. Use 5–10 drops of Reckeweg **R1** every 3 hours and 10 drops of Reckeweg **R4** 3 times daily. In chronic problems with associated weakness, take 15 drops of Reckeweg R26 once daily. Ask the chemist to advise you on taking an electrolyte replacement as well. Drink tea made from dulse – a seaweed gathered from the west coast of Scotland – and Irish Moss and carrageen.

Try using a positive thought for stimulating your excretory system.

'I am safe to let go of all my past pain, hurt and poisonous waste, physically, emotionally and spiritually.'

The Digestive System

PHASE THREE

```
    3
  EARTH
   taste
 Sugars and
carbohydrates
```

For guidance on how to use the information in this section see p. 65.

For guidance on how to use the information in this section see p. 65.

To discuss the stomach and digestive system we must first talk about hunger. There must be the presence of 'real' physical hunger for food to be properly assimilated into the system. Ask yourself whether you eat because you are hungry or out of habit, boredom, or some psychological need or pain. Without real hunger, food that goes into the stomach and digestive tract will not be broken down effectively and this may well create problems.

Once food enters the mouth a series of enzymes are released to break food down for assimilation and absorption from the bowel and intestines into the bloodstream, then on to nourish all the cells of the body. The word 'enzyme' comes from the Greek word 'enzymos', meaning life-giving. Some enzymes break down carbohydrates (starch), others break down fats, and still others, proteins.

The stomach senses and weighs up the food (both literally and figuratively) and receives information from the hypothalamus and pituitary (which direct the salivary glands, stomach, pancreas and intestines). Inside the stomach gastric juices are secreted to continue the process, rather like 'stoking the fire'. The resulting 'chyme' moves through the duodenum and is broken down into smaller units of energy under the control of the liver and pancreas. The pancreas keeps track of all the enzymes required, and releases insulin; the adrenal glands secrete minerals and hormones. Inside the intestines the hair-like fibres that undulate (rather like a car wash operates to clean your car) absorb nutrients in their simplest form. Anything that is not broken down passes through and is formed into faeces.

The digestive system reacts sympathetically to all kinds of stress, which reduces its capacity to function. When the body, mind and spirit experience negative influences such as worry, anxiety and fear, food sits in the digestive system very heavily, turning into waste that poisons the body and effectively causes starvation on a cellular level. Many people today in affluent Western societies are eating the wrong kinds of food and this produces problems of malabsorption. The pollution and toxic waste materials from industry also upset the stomach and the digestive system, which in turn destroys the vitality of the liver. Junk foods and any commercially processed food creates an imbalance of stress in the body, giving rise to digestive disorders resulting from acid–alkaline imbalances. The use of antacids, most of which contain aluminium, gives rise to addictive habits, without any resolution of the real problem. A weak and polluted digestive system sets the stage for the degeneration of the vital organs; the liver, pancreas, heart, kidneys and spleen. The sweet flavour that the Chinese and Oriental sages understood was the taste of the stomach and its sympathetic response and reaction to everything around it in the environment. They recognised that the being who was no longer 'singing a happy song' was in danger of becoming sour from a sad liver and unhappy from the stomach. The mouth would then begin to turn down instead of turning up from habitual happiness. The affected digestive juices and fluids would create the desire to get rid of the contaminated foods that were upsetting the emotional and physical states of balance. How wise they were! When there are symptoms such as heartburn, gas, wind, belching, flatulence, sore tongue and bad breath, this is a sign that the digestive tract/stomach is being 'beaten up' and losing the battle against badly chosen foods and the polluted environment. Healing treatment is needed. When the enzymes of fruits, vegetables, grains, beans and meats are eaten in the right proportions (see the diet plans on p. 41), the body will look, feel and smell good, and have the desires that nature designed it for! Constant bloating, rumbling and grumbling are the signs that the inner being is rebelling against poisonous foods. The order of the day is new foods, and a new lifestyle free from so much stress.

Make sure that you are exercising regularly. Walking and swimming are the best. Avoid jogging and cycling. Do some yoga. Learn how to relax. Make sure that you take at least 5 minutes to calm down before eating.

FOODS

To support the stomach and the digestive system, increase the vegetables in both Phase One and Phase Two referring to the Five Phase food chart (see p. 170). Reduce the grains and beans of Phase One – wheat, oats, rye and barley – as this will 'pierce' the Earth Phase. Eat millet at least once every day. Avoid bread, cheese, cream, butter, tomatoes, peppers, oranges, grapefruit, rhubarb, peanuts, brazil nuts, cashews (these nuts are too fatty and hard on an already weakened digestion), mayonnaise, salad cream, shellfish, coffee, tea, alcohol, white flour, white sugar, all junk foods, cooked oils and fried foods like chips and crisps. Reduce your consumption of butter. Do not eat too many pulses as they are hard to digest. If you must eat them, cook them very well with fresh ginger and thyme. Take live acidophilus yoghurt and water every day 15 minutes after meals (2 teaspoons of yoghurt stirred into a glass of water).

SUPPLEMENTS

For acute problems with the stomach and digestion, take 2 capsules of acidophilus after each meal and 1,000mg of pantothenic acid. This stimulates the metabolism of fats, proteins and carbohydrates. Take 1 capsule of a digestive enzyme (see *Resources*) after your main meal. These are the 2 most important supplements for conditions of the stomach. For wind, gas or cramps take 3 tablets of magnesium phosphate under the tongue every 4–6 hours, or the multiple formula tissue salts for dyspepsia–indigestion, 2 tablets dissolved under the tongue every 2–3 hours, and 1 capsule of the Bio-Care Ligazyme formula after each meal.

Reckeweg R1 (inflammation drops) and R5 (stomach drops), 10 drops should be taken every 4–6 hours until there is an improvement. Take R92 (digestive enzyme formula), 20–30 drops half an hour after the main meal.

For chronic problems, take 1 capsule of **acidophilus** after meals; 1 capsule of **pantothenic acid** after breakfast and lunch; 3 tablets of magnesium phosphate 3 times daily under the tongue; 1 capsule of Bio-Care's Digest-aid after your main meal; 1 multivitamin capsule after breakfast or lunch; 3 tablets of iron phosphate (Ferr. Phos.) tissue salt under the tongue 3 times daily, 1 hour after meals; and 1,000mg of vitamin C daily (as calcium or magnesium ascorbate). Also use Reckeweg R1 and **R5**; 10 drops 3 times daily; and R92, 20 drops after lunch and dinner.

Try using a positive thought for stimulating your digestive system.

'I am digesting and assimilating all my food; I am satisfied and nourished.'

GROUP 5

The Sinus, Ears, Nose and Throat

PHASE TWO

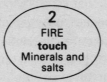

2
FIRE
touch
Minerals and
salts

For guidance on how to use the information in this section see p. 65.

The hypothalamus and the pituitary gland plan and arrange all the decisions for the battle and war when under attack. The anterior pituitary regulates the entire commitment of forces or 'energy' production in the body via the thyroid. The thyroid regulates the overall metabolism of foods under the direct power of the adrenal glands.

The anterior pituitary also deals with sex hormones via the adrenal glands. When you become exhausted, the hormone balance between the pituitary and adrenals is disturbed and the processes that they regulate do not function properly. One of the most important functions of the pituitary is the control of the stages of growth through the release of the growth hormone. This is coordinated from the time of conception, as the foetus develops, and through the entire life process from infancy to maturity. The pituitary accomplishes the hormonal activity of all physical development. Environmental changes directly affect the pituitary, opposing the natural unfolding of genetic Life Energy. Environmental poisons, especially the heavy metals from industrial waste, and nuclear radiation, can and I believe are causing mutations within the genetic material of our species. Down's Syndrome and other birth defects are due in part to the cellular poisoning from toxins that are subtly and profoundly affecting our 'blueprint' for living.

The Ancient Indian (Vedic) tradition prescribed meditation, Hatha Yoga, and other physical and spiritual practices to stimulate and unlock the powers of the body (in the form of chemical hormones) to stay youthful forever. I am certain that one of the reasons that so many people are turning to the ways of the East is because they feel there may be helpful ways to resolve the dilemma of health problems today and to improve the quality of life, rather than try to extend the length of it by any chemical means necessary. The ancient sages believed that the pituitary could unlock the power to see beyond normal reality. Individuals could learn to transport their bodies in 'astral travel' and observe anything, anywhere, anytime, at will. Through this power individuals could 'think' a thought and have complete control over every physical sense, and thus be masters of their own destiny. Through the physical world they could accomplish anything they wanted. There are still such sages in India, apparently.

Through the senses the pituitary receives 'data' from the environment and readjusts its chemical stance via the adrenal glands. Fear and courage are regulated through the pituitary. With the stress, pressure, pace and poisons in our environment today we have collectively created a situation that thwarts our ability to feel safe and comfortable as opposed to fearful and trapped.

As well as controlling ageing, the anterior pituitary is affected by pressure changes. For example, when stormy weather approaches and the barometric pressure plummets, the pituitary registers this and readjusts the level of acidity by increasing it in the whole of the body, especially the area in the head where the ears, nose and throat meet. Chinese medicine takes these 'sacred spaces' into account. They are as important as the glands and organs. Our present modern medicine has no concept of 'spaces' inside the body being in balance with the 'solid' glands and organs. The focus of treatment in the West takes only the physical into account; it does not see the body as sacred or in any sense spiritual. It is just a replaceable mechanical machine with interchangeable parts. Doctors, most especially surgeons, should be required to learn from their forebears, the great Chinese and Indian sages! The ancient and modern, East and West, need to be integrated to confront the profound challenges of our time.

Creation has placed great responsibility on the pituitary to adapt to the changes in our environment. We must take responsibility for our lives and this begins with caring for our physical and emotional health. To look to someone else to tell you what to do is not practical.

Physical conditions that manifest as a result of pituitary imbalance include sinus troubles, blocked ears, nose or throat sensations (or pains), colds, flu, coughs, excessive dryness, excessive catarrh, tickle in the throat, ringing in the ears. Problems may also arise with the pituitary because of excessive quantities of hormones – or too few – being secreted by the pituitary. This can cause fluid problems, such as swollen hands, face or feet. Hereditary defects of the pituitary require careful diagnosis as well as a plan for treatment that integrates the doctor's advice with a nutritional approach. This minimises the need for long-term specialist support and emphasises instead the life-giving qualities of a balanced diet.

FOODS
The following dietary adjustments will aid the recovery of the pituitary, sinus, ears, nose and throat. Eat more Phase One vegetables, particularly dark, leafy greens and carrots, broccoli, green beans and green peas. Eat more corn porridge (polenta) and asparagus. Eat more Phase Two vegetables, grains, fruits, nuts and seeds. Yoghurt is also very good. Reduce wheat, oats, rye, butter, cream, beer, coffee, tea, tobacco, wine and chocolate.

SUPPLEMENTS

Vitamin C is very helpful for all types of sinus problems. In acute cases take 1,000mg every 3–4 hours; for chronic conditions, take 1,000mg 3–4 times a day. Calcium or magnesium ascorbate provides the best source of this vitamin. Take vitamin A in the form of beta-carotene in acute cases, 25,000i.u. once or twice daily for 7–10 days. If the problem is chronic, take 25,000i.u. once daily for at least a month. Use only the water-soluble vitamin, or liquid vitamin A (see *Resources*). Use Bee Propolis capsules, in acute cases 2 capsules 3–4 times a day for 2–4 weeks; for chronic conditions, 1 or 2 capsules daily for at least 2–3 months. Take dry succinate vitamin E in acute cases, 400i.u. twice daily; for chronic conditions, 400–800i.u. daily for alternate months for 6 months.

Take elemental zinc in acute cases, 50mg 3 times per day; for chronic cases, 30mg twice a day for 3–4 months. Take the herb Echinacea as a liquid (see *Resources*), in acute cases, 20–30 drops in water every 3–6 hours for 5 days. In chronic cases, take 20 drops twice daily for 2–3 months.

Reckeweg homeopathic remedies are also useful here. **R1** for inflammation, in acute cases 10 drops every 4–6 hours for alternate 7 day periods for 1 month. For chronic cases, 10 drops 3 times a day for 1 month. Use R93 for a weak immune system that may accompany sinus troubles. Take it with R1, 10 drops 3 times daily in acute cases; or on its own, 10 drops every 3–4 hours for 7 days. For chronic cases take 10 drops 3 times a day for 2–3 weeks. For catarrh and sinusitis, take R49, 10 drops every 2–3 hours for 3 days, in acute cases; for chronic conditions take 10 drops 3 times a day for 3 weeks.

Try using a positive thought for stimulating your anterior pituitary.

'I am enjoying being in control of my body mind and spirit.'

GROUP 6

The Liver
and Gall Bladder

PHASE ONE

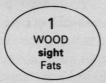

1
WOOD
sight
Fats

For guidance on how to use the information in this section see p. 65.

When Group 6 is in either your first or last group in your test results, it means you have an imbalance within your liver and gall bladder. The liver is the largest organ in the body; it regulates the absorption of foods, mixing numerous enzymes with food from the intestines to aid metabolism. The liver makes the food ready for transportation to all cells for use, and the rest is held in storage for the future. The liver is the major organ of 'purification'. It increases the 'aliveness' of the blood hence its name 'live-r'! The health of the liver reflects and reveals the ageing or youthful quality of the whole body. The organ has a self-rejuvenating capacity; for example if it is damaged by disease such as cirrhosis, due to excessive alcohol consumption, the liver can restore damaged tissue once alcohol consumption stops. This indicates an evolutionary biological link to the past with sea creatures and amphibians which also regenerate lost body mass.

The liver regulates the metabolism of fats, proteins and carbohydrates. The organ's main function is its unique position in a triad between the adrenal glands and pancreas for the blood sugar metabolism. The liver and the gall bladder (which regulates the movement of bile for fat metabolism) can become

extremely toxic from absorbing poisons from the environment. When other vital areas of the body become sick or
diseased the liver tries to take over the function and
demands. The liver contains all the genetic programmes for
every possible combination of amino acids to make proteins
laid down through the life blueprint from the start of
evolution. The liver is affected by changes in the acid–
alkaline balance. When the body is affected physically or
emotionally by heavy metal poisoning in the external environment, the liver tries to balance the carbon–nitrogen cycle in
the body. All addiction to substances, whether sugar, alcohol, tobacco or hard drugs, will destroy the liver. The liver
gives life in the form of energy – sugar – for the body.

When the liver is sick, a sour taste and 'sour' feelings are
present. Fats remain undigested inside the body and turn
rancid. The eyes lose their sparkle and the face looks
yellowy-green. The individual will get angry to conceal deep
sadness. Shouting will hide tears. The winds will make the
eyes water; the vision may become poor, and the neck will
feel extremely tense and 'sour', particularly on the right side.
The nails will become spotted, fungus may grow on the
fingers and toes. The shoulders will slope around the heart,
looking as if they are carrying the problems of the world. The
muscles will stiffen as tight as a board. Decision making will
be difficult and particularly reading will become progressively
more laboured and confusing. Heaviness after eating breakfast will put sufferers off their foods; then they may eat like a
hungry dog, waking in the middle of the night with a sour
upset tummy and pains on the right side of the lower
abdomen. The mouth will carry the taste of metal. This will
be worse when they wake from sleep.

FOODS
When the above symptoms become a problem, try making the
following dietary adjustments. Eat lots of fresh, raw and cooked
greens from all the Phases (see the Five Phase food chart on p.

170), especially broccoli, green beans, carrots, peas and globe artichokes, which should be taken cooked not raw. Also helpful are watercress, parsley, dark green lettuce, chard, mustard and cress, endive, escarole, chicory, green onions, courgettes, celery, chinese cabbage, turnip greens, mustard greens, curly kale. Raw salads are good once a day, preferably at lunch. All these greens will help break down the bile which may become congested when the liver is sad and unwell. Like cures like and green foods support the liver because they are high in enzymes, which are the natural 'detergents' which can clean up the bloodstream and fluids of the body.

Avoid all the acid foods; tomatoes, peppers, aubergine, spinach, oranges, grapefruit, all pulses, peanuts, brazil, cashew and pistachio nuts, wheat and oats. Steer clear of butter, cream, salad cream and mayonnaise. Increase the Phase Five foods, especially buckwheat, sea vegetables, beets, beet greens, berries. During the summer months eat watermelon in the morning by itself to help cleanse the liver and gall bladder. Upon rising drink water and lemon every day, adding increasing amounts of cayenne pepper. Use the African grown cayenne if possible, but only a tiny pinch, because this pepper is the hottest in the world. Make a pâté from chicken livers and a little lemon and olive oil, to help the liver restore the metabolism and, particularly, protein absorption. Most people have difficulty digesting pulses. Therefore, if there are any liver symptoms it is best to avoid split peas and lentils. Avoid sour pickles, sauerkraut and all vinegars (with the exception of a little balsamic vinegar). Very strong cravings for sour foods will be reduced by eating the Phase One vegetables. Do not eat yeast products such as Marmite, Vegemite, Vecon or any other concentrated salt. Use miso made from barley sparingly instead of salt. Breads should be eaten 2–3 times a week at the most. Avoid ham, pork, luncheon meats or smoked meats.

SUPPLEMENTS
Of single most importance when treating the liver is to detoxify it of waste and poisons as quickly as possible, yet without

causing a healing crisis, in which the body becomes feverish, cold and has flu symptoms, diarrhoea, headaches, physical and emotional disorientation as the whole system improves. Choline, inositol, vitamin E, selenium, methionine, cysteine, cystine, all are anti-oxidants that can help restore normal liver functions when they are poisoned by waste from foods, the environment, addictions, emotional shocks and traumas.

Bio-Care company formulas: Cell-guard, Hep-194, Oxyplex and Ligazyme, can be taken for a period of thirty days. Cell-guard and Hep-194 are specifically targeted to the liver pathways, stimulating the release of undigested bile salts, fats and heavy metals stored in the liver. Take 1 capsule of each at lunch and dinner. Take Oxyplex only at breakfast time, once a day. Take 1 capsule of Ligazyme 3 times daily. Ligazyme provides vital B vitamins and minerals to maintain tissue during detoxification. In cases where high levels of low density lipids or high cholesterol have been diagnosed by a doctor or other health practitioner, take 1 capsule of phosphitidyl choline twice a day. Green Magma, a product from Japan made from sprouted young organic barley can be taken twice a day to detoxify the liver; 1 teaspoon stirred into a glass of water. A mixture of carrot, celery, beet and watercress juices will also help detoxify the liver. Make a drink from 2 carrots, 2 stalks of celery, 1 raw peeled beetroot and a quarter of a bunch of watercress, a juice combination based on the recommendations of the famous naturopath–hygienist Norman Walker, an octogenarian American. Digestive enzymes betaine hydrochloride and comfrey pepsin can be taken at lunch and dinner.

Take Reckeweg **R7**, liver/gall bladder drops, for calculi, stones, constipation, bile troubles or lack of appetite. For acute cases, 10 drops every 3–4 hours; chronic conditions require 15 drops twice daily. For severe congestion use R26, Draining Stimulating drops, or R60 Blood Purifying drops can be taken alternately every other day; in acute cases, 15 drops twice daily; for chronic conditions, 10 drops 3 times daily.

The herbs **Ginko Biloba** and Gota Kola can be taken 1

month later. Take 1 capsule of each daily over 3 months to help restore the liver functions gently.

Try using a positive thought for stimulating your liver.

'I am rejuvenating my body, mind and spirit to keep in balance and live life to the fullest of my human potential.'

GROUP 7

The Lungs and Respiratory System
PHASE FOUR

$$\left(\begin{array}{c} 4 \\ \text{METAL} \\ \textbf{smell} \\ \text{Amino acids} \end{array}\right)$$

For guidance on how to use the information in this section see p. 65.

For guidance on how to use the information in this section see p. 65.

When Group 7 appears as the first or last number in your analysis, it means that your breathing and related conditions are out of balance.

Every chemical process in the body depends on the breath. The routine of the breath sets the rhythm of the circulatory as well as the cardiovascular system. The lungs cannot be separated from the heart. The monotonous rhythm of the breath creates an engine-like rise and fall, the contracting and relaxing movement of the heart. Each breath contains approximately $3\frac{1}{2}$ movements of the pulse. Through the movement of the pulse, the Chinese are able to record how well the body is functioning.

Every part of the body, from the most solid organs to the space of the cavities, can be poisoned by what is absorbed from the external environment. During the exchange of oxygen and carbon dioxide, the lungs supply vitally important nutrients via the red blood cells, through the pumping action of the heart. Every negative condition that affects the body is reflected in the changing movement of the breathing and therefore in the changing supply of fresh nutrients. Constricted breathing is the biochemical response to stress. The effects of stress and air pollution on the body are causing allergies (such as hay fever), bronchitis, asthma, emphysema and severe respiratory imbalances. Pollution may also cause catarrh, coughs, sore throats, and general irritation and inflammation to the mucous membranes.

In Chinese medicine there is the understanding of the inseparable link between the lungs and the nose. Lung problems are always accompanied by disturbances in the nasal fluids. Too much or too little mucus flows because of external irritants. Too little mucus makes the body overheat, causing dryness on the skin's surface. Both conditions can exist together or swing from one to the other.

The Oriental doctor also understands the importance of the thyroid and the regulation of minerals transported through the lungs, which controls a large part of the metabolism. Disrupted breathing prevents the heart and hence the energy of the whole body from functioning efficiently. The rhythm of the body and all its processes is lost.

Proteins are the most important building block of nourishment for the lungs. They guarantee the continual rebuilding of new cells. When the body is invaded and its defence penetrated due to 'foreign' substances infiltrating the inside surfaces of the lungs, the body may try to force it out by coughing. When the body is over-run with poisonous waste it may attempt to thwart the harmful invaders by wheezing, constriction and coughing. These are symptoms of asthma, which may appear as the body tries to throw out the toxic waste that is literally strangling it. The laboured breathing of an asthmatic is extremely painful to witness and can be life-threatening to its victim. ALL ASTHMATICS ARE CARRYING AN EXCESS LOAD OF PHYSICAL AND EMOTIONAL WASTE! The use of breathing stimulants, such as Ventolin and Becotide, to help the breathing can only work in the short term. Their ongoing use creates addiction and dependency and further weakens the underlying imbalances! The continual use of steroids cannot tackle the underlying toxaemia that is creating the problems: rather, it eventually destroys the energy system, the bones and the muscles!

Detoxification is the answer to lung disorders. In all cases the possibility of infection in the chest and lung cavity must be investigated. Pneumonia, and various bacterial and viral diseases must be diagnosed. Poisons that have established themselves in the lungs, bronchials or pleura must be ejected quickly in order to protect the body. Suppressive drugs destroy the body's own ability to protect itself and must only be used as a last resort, not as a first choice of treatment.

FOODS
To support the work of the lungs, eat more of the Phase Three foods: millet, sweet potatoes, yams, artichokes, yellow squash and corn on the cob. Also eat more Phase Four vegetables: cabbage, cauliflower, celery, chinese cabbage, leeks, radish and watercress. Refer to the Five Phase food chart on p. 170 and decrease Phase Four grains and beans: rice, potato and soya beans. Increase Phase Three beans: chick peas. Increase Phase Three fruits: apples, bananas, mango, papaya, pineapple. Increase Phase Four fruits: peaches and pears. Increase Phase Three nuts and seeds: almonds, hazeluts and pine nuts. Avoid walnuts, which are Phase Four nuts. Avoid all dairy products except for yoghurt. All cheeses are to be avoided. Increase your fish consumption, choosing from Phase Three and Phase Four. Avoid beef and turkey, but increase quail and pheasant. Avoid all sweets: carob, honey, sugar, brown or white. Avoid all soy products.

SUPPLEMENTS
Take a good **multivitamin** and **multimineral** every day (see *Resources*). Vitamin C is useful in every lung-related disorder. Massive doses can be used instead of steroids. Vitamin C in such doses works as a natural antibiotic, and so does Bee Propolis, Golden Seal, garlic and Echinacea. This combination will fight off bacteria. Vitamins A and E and zinc will help

stimulate and activate the enfeebled immune system. Pantothenic acid must be used in order to stimulate the energy system. Use it with L-Methionine, choline and inositol, which together help to break down concentrated waste in the form of heavy, sticky mucus.

For acute lung or general respiratory problems, use Reckeweg formula R1. Take 10 drops every 3 hours for acute problems; for chronic conditions 10 drops in half a glass of water 3–4 times a day. For bronchitis, whooping cough, and irritations of the upper air passages, take R9 drops. In acute cases, 10 drops every 2–3 hours; for chronic conditions 10 drops in half a glass of water 3–4 times a day. For bronchial congestion or catarrh, take R48. In acute cases take 10 drops every 3–4 hours; for chronic conditions 10 drops in half a glass of water 3–4 times a day. For asthma, take R43. In acute cases 10 drops every 1–2 hours; for chronic conditions, 10 drops, 3–6 times a day.

Try using a positive thought for stimulating your lungs.

'I am breathing fresh, purified air for my whole body, mind and spirit to be constantly refreshed.'

GROUP 8

The Sex Organs and the Reproductive System

PHASE ONE

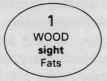

1
WOOD
sight
Fats

For guidance on how to use the information in this section see p. 65.

When Group 8 appears in the analysis of your test, it indicates a disturbance or the beginnings of a disease affecting the reproductive system. In the female system this could be affecting the uterus, the ovaries, vagina, or the womb itself. In the male system the penis, scrotum or testes may be involved. Much has been written about the reproductive system, yet it is the most misunderstood area of the human body.

The reproductive system and the sex organs are located very close to the elimination system. Creation and decay therefore reside in the same area of the body. However, their activities are mutually exclusive; sexual activity stops the 'letting go' of waste matter so that the flow and reception of semen from the male to the female can take place and potentially create new life. Children begin their independence from their parents by taking control of the elimination organs during 'potty training'. The problems that can arise during this process may wound a child psychologically. It may take a lifetime to heal the disturbance to the process of 'letting go' or 'surrendering', which is also vital in the act of making love. Letting go of waste matter, and letting go to receive love are very closely linked physically, emotionally and psychologically. Any problems connected with this area are stored and may rise to the surface during the act of making love, so disturbing the 'biological release' of orgasm that should bring ecstatic pleasure to every human being.

If the sex organs themselves have been violated or abused physically or emotionally before an individual is naturally sexually active, the individual in question often acts out unconsciously and uncontrollably a self-destructive drive, and may also be destructive to another. This area of the body causes more physical and emotional human suffering than anywhere else in our bodies. No other area of the body can individually or collectively reflect the human confusion and misunderstanding of the design and potential of our Life Energy. Wilheim Reich, the famous colleague of Sigmund Freud, devoted his entire life to understanding human suffering and human aggression which arose from sexuality. His main premise was that human beings have a biological need to 'release' during love-making, through orgasm. Any anxiety, neuroses or psychosis would damage and reduce this potential. He further believed that all diseases were rooted in the reduction of this energy he called Orgone, another name for Life Energy. In simple terms, Reich recognised how the whole modern social processes at work in capitalism and socialism suppressed, repressed, depressed, compressed and oppressed the individual body, mind and spirit in order to maintain the status quo. In doing so it disempowered the human being. Reich was attacked for his revolutionary ideas by the established medical community in America, as well as the Food and Drug Administration under the control of the massive drug companies. Reich's work helped free me from my 'rock' of suffering that came from the emotional and physical abuse that I suffered from both my parents as a child. It helped save my life and restore my humanity.

Through the biological function of the sex organs we energetically work towards balancing our positive and negative, male and female energies. In simple terms the male, Yang energy is a 'giving', radiant energy and the female, Yin energy is a 'receiving' energy. These two forces make the duality that moves Life

Energy through the entire physical universe. The two energies are not separate! The historical conditioning that has made us separate our ideas of male–female, positive–negative, push–pull, radiation-gravitation, spirit–matter, mother–father has separated us from our other halves. The modern traditions surrounding the birth process create the beginnings of this separation. The trauma of a violent birth promotes unconscious wounds, trauma, shock, injury, at physical, emotional and spiritual levels. Our birth experience works at the level of the unconscious and establishes the way we think about the world. If this prevents us from experiencing unity of male and female and the healthy expression of giving and receiving in the act of love-making, we are sowing the seeds of destruction in society! Men and women must be able to trust each other to provide a unity; a balance of male and female. The reproductive system and the sex organs carry all the memories of birth as well as unconscious fears of death. Birth is the female principle and death is the male principle. They cannot be separated! The basic physical law of the entire universe is unity-oneness! By accepting the connectedness of male and female, we can share our human potential fully through the act of love.

Problems with the reproductive system and sex organs are a sign of unresolved physical or emotional abuse. This will almost always initially be denied by the individual who is troubled. The main treatment is to talk out one's 'story'. No other treatment is more vital to heal any sickness in this area because it so much relates to what we really feel about ourselves. Self-deprecation, and not feeling good enough in all sorts of ways, goes hand in hand with imbalances in the reproductive system and sex organs. Anyone consulting a practitioner for treatment needs strong psychological support. A wholistic approach is critical for problems in this area.

FOODS
The foods that support the sex organs are the Phase Five foods. Refer to the Five Phase food chart on p. 170. All the

'water' foods support the 'conception' and 'birth-creation' foods of the Wood phase (see chart, p. 168). The sex organs, which are part of Phase One, are supported by all the green foods. Proteins are the most important for the maturation of healthy sex organs. To rebuild and strengthen the sex organs and reproductive system, eat proteins that the body can absorb easily. It is absolutely necessary that the proteins match the individual's chemistry. Otherwise, a variety of problems can ensue, such as (for women), PMT, endometriosis, ovarian growth, tumours or breast inflammation. For men, there could be a prostate condition or a virility problem. These imbalances can develop further into cancerous growth due to irregularities in the metabolism of protein. Broccoli, all kinds of green lettuces, parsley, green peas, string beans, courgettes and carrots are helpful to support the sex organs and reproductive system. Eat less wheat, oats, rye and barley because these grains are acid-forming and weaken the sex organs and reproductive system. All Phase Five grains and beans support the sex organs and reproductive system, especially buckwheat groats (kasha), and soba noodles, Japanese pasta. Sea vegetables are an important protein for the sex organs and reproductive system because they contain the full spectrum of amino acids plus all of the essential micro-nutrients. Sperm and other bodily fluids have chemical properties similar to many types of sea life. Fish protein is very supportive for healthy functioning sex organs because it is high in zinc, vitamin E, calcium, potassium, manganese, magnesium and sulphur.

SUPPLEMENTS
For any disturbances affecting the reproductive system you need a multivitamin (see *Resources*). For gynaecological problems of any type women may take Dong Quai (angelica). This is a herb that tones the entire female reproductive system and gives support to the elasticity of all mucous membrane and soft tissue. It is most effective taken with

calcium and magnesium which are used up during menstruation, potentially setting the stage for bone and muscle
troubles: osteoporosis, rheumatoid arthritis, callouses, foot
troubles. Take 500mg calcium at least once a day. The best
type of calcium is the EAP form. Vitamin B6 can be taken
with any multiple formula; in fact it should not be taken
separately. Always use the Pyridoxyl–5–Phosphate form of
B6, which is more easily absorbed and utilised by the body.
Magnesium EAP is the best form of this mineral to ingest.
Like calcium EAP, magnesium supports all nerve, muscle and
soft tissue. Magnesium works with calcium to counterbalance
the push towards acidity.

For hormone balance and support all the unsaturated fatty
acids are vital. **GLA** is the most important oil because it
directly helps balance the pituitary, from which many reproductive hormones are released into the body. They, in turn,
stimulate the thyroid gland, and this works on the energy
cycle via the adrenals and pancreas. Problems with the
reproductive system always manifest a corresponding energy
imbalance that affects blood sugar levels. Fatigue, lethargy,
sleeplessness, nervousness, hysteria and overwhelming
emotional states are all symptoms of an imbalanced energy
system.

The homeopathic formula **R20**, from Reckeweg, is important
when this group appears in your questionnaire result. This
supports the whole female system or 'circuit'. Take 10 drops in
half a glass of water 3 times a day, first upon rising, then half an
hour before dinner, and then before bed.

For male problems with the reproductive system, all the
above recommendations apply except the Dong Quai. Men
can take 500mg Ginseng, 1–3 times a day. I recommend Red
Tien Ginseng as the best tonic for virility or potency
problems, prostate, bladder and other ailments of the male
system. **Vitamin E** can be supplemented with up to 600i.u.
of d-alpha tocopherol (the natural strain of utilisable vitamin
E). Reckeweg's formula **R19** supports the male system.

Take 15 drops twice daily in half a glass of water, upon rising
and before bed.

Try using a positive thought for stimulating your reproductive
system.

'I am attracting and creating a perfect balance, a positive and
negative, male and female energies that support my sexuality
and sensuality.'

GROUP 9

The Skeletal
and Muscular Systems

PHASE FIVE

5
WATER
hearing
Water

For guidance on how to use the information in this section see p.65.

'The power of the body is exerted by the muscles, which represent the love of work in the mind, and in the spirit . . . The least living parts of the body are the bones, which are composed largely of earthly material, and seem to have a use like that of the rocks in nature; that is, they serve as a basic fulcrum for the softer parts, keeping them extended in their right places, and serving also as protection to the organs that specifically need protection. The rocks, and likewise the bones, correspond to fixed facts upon which all the other elements of mental life depend; . . . holding firmly to certain facts of experience . . .'

Physiological Correspondences, John Worcester, 1889.

When Group 9 appears in your questionnaire results, it means that an imbalance is developing in your bones and muscles. This may range from simple tensions, strains and stresses, to degenerative bone diseases. When life experiences stress the physical structure of the human body, there is a tendency to contract the muscles causing the physical or emotional pain to be stored. Under such tension, breathing is restricted, holding and trapping negative physical energy in sympathy with the rest of the body. This creates acidity in the muscle tissue. A high level of acidity 'shuts off' nerve response and holds the pain and hurt. At the same time it creates a tendency to blame oneself and not feel 'good enough'. Over time this represses and suppresses the individual. As a consequence their movements become restricted, jerky, limited and tense. The body loses its vitality and receptivity to respond positively and becomes a 'limited' expression of the personality. Anyone with bone and muscle trouble has unresolved traumas from the past that are being stored inside the body. This is also true of injuries that continue to plague an individual. All conditions affecting the bones and muscles are caused by the flow of poisons in the form of uric acid through the lymph stream. The bones were used by the ancients to 'read' the past and prophesy the future. A Canadian dentist found that he could read the baby teeth and know precisely by the colour and the calcium layer the emotional and physical traumas the child had endured before the age of 6. The accuracy of his readings astounded his colleagues!

Western clinical analysis and Eastern 'oracle' almost appear to meet at this point. Western medicine might yet re-learn the skills of diagnosing imbalances and disease from the 'story' that is revealed by a single part of the body.

Extreme acidity affects the relationship of the energy system to the digestive system. The absorption of foods is hampered, and the bones and muscles begin to be overwhelmed by the undigested fats, proteins and carbohydrates that are stored as waste in the body. This sets the stage for many of the degenerative diseases of the bones and muscles. Acidity can manifest itself and deposit excess waste in any part of the body, depending on the biochemical weakness of the individual. This in turn, depends on climate and the environment and genetic factors. Most importantly, such weaknesses arise as a result of the physiological effect of the foods eaten. Acidity is always accompanied by fluid retention, swelling, pain, redness and changes in skin tone. All of these tend to increase the ageing process. Too much acid in the acid–alkaline balance is registered first in the body's muscles and the bones. It is experienced as muscular contraction and tension. If arthritis develops, it produces inflammation or infection. There are several varieties of arthritis and rheumatism which are the result of excess acidity that leads to excess uric acid being deposited throughout the joints. Rheumatism will usually become a chronic disease; the excess acidity changes the structure of the joints, 'burning up' the vital fluids that lubricate the joints. In extreme cases the joints are deformed by this and can give the sufferer a great deal of pain. All of these conditions are brought on by acidity which is like 'fire' burning the tissue. If the immune system cannot cope, the degenerative conditions become established. Stretching and yoga exercises stimulate the glands and organs, and help to drain the lymph glands.

Loss of bone calcium is a major problem resulting from excess acidity, which in turn is the result of pressure, stress, incorrect dietary intake, and hormonal and energy problems. Women's health is under threat because the environment is 'stealing' minerals from their bodies, increasing the risk of bone softening.

FOODS

Food plays a very important role in the treatment of bone and muscle problems. Since acidity disturbs the work of the body's enzymes, it prevents digestion, absorption, assimilation and elimination, so undermining the efficiency of fats, proteins and carbohydrates in the diet. Congestion may build up in the lymphatic systems, preventing the body from getting rid of waste.

Foods to avoid include acid-forming vegetables, fruit and grains such as red and green peppers, oats, spinach, oranges and grapefruit. Decrease wheat consumption and eat yeasted wheat bread only occasionally. Reduce your intake of peanuts, cashews, cheese, ice cream, sour cream, cream, salad cream, pistachios and shellfish (other than prawns). Keep tea and coffee consumption to a maximum of 3 cups of either, daily. Red meat and pork should only be eaten once or twice weekly, if at all. Vinegar, pickles and sauerkraut, may be eaten occasionally. Eat a balanced diet, taken from all Phases in the Five Phase food chart on p. 170.

SUPPLEMENTS

Take a multivitamin with a range of B vitamins. Increase your mineral consumption with 250mg **magnesium EAP** and **calcium EAP**. Supplement these with Devil's Claw, a herb taken in capsule form 1–3 times a day. Vitamin C in the form of calcium ascorbate and magnesium ascorbate will help break down toxins and acidity, and drain the lymph glands. Digestive enzymes should be taken with lunch and dinner (see *Resources*). Vitamin B5, pantothenic acid, is helpful to stimulate the adrenal glands and reduce joint inflammation. Take 500–1,000mg with breakfast and lunch.

From the Reckeweg homeopathic remedies, take R1 for inflammation and infection, R46 for arthritis, with R11 for muscular or joint pain in the arms, fingers, hips and back. Take the remedies twice daily, 15 drops in half a glass of water upon rising and again before bed.

Try using a positive thought for stimulating your skeletal and muscular systems.

'I am letting go of all my personal history and from holding the past against me.'

GROUP 10

The Thyroid Gland and Metabolism

PHASE FOUR

4
METAL
smell
Amino acids

For guidance on how to use the information in this section see page 65.

When the thyroid appears as the first (box A) or second number (box B) questionnaire analysis, it indicates that there are patterned imbalances affecting the ability to metabolise food and regulate the whole energy conversion cycle within the body. The thyroid controls the action of all physical processes in the body. Located in and around the Adam's apple, the thyroid is the most exposed gland of the entire body apart from the sex organs, which are normally covered by clothing. The thyroid receives information from the hypothalamus and pituitary glands. This arrives in the form of a surge of electrical energy (with a corresponding increase in pressure). The thyroid then secretes and mixes minerals, which are sent to the pancreas, adrenal glands and liver. All these are part of the energy system. When the thyroid is out of balance, the possibility increases of having anxiety attacks, panic attacks, or experiencing loss of confidence, weakness, helplessness or powerlessness. In extreme cases it may cause neurotic, schizophrenic and even psychotic behaviour.

I believe that the anti-social and sometimes violent behaviour of criminals may be due to biochemical imbalances that may be rooted in glandular disturbances of the thyroid. These imbalances make the body react with pathological behaviour, and are triggered by eating nutritionally deficient foods, lacking in the vital vitamins and minerals that the thyroid gland needs. When the thyroid is out of balance it may become difficult for certain individuals to cope, and to distinguish between 'good' and 'evil'. Delusions and paranoia may result from the body, mind and spirit experiencing the stresses and strains of everyday living, coupled with the threat of poisons from the environment.

Thyroid imbalance and disease make chemical activity in the thyroid either excessive or insufficient. Vertigo, dizziness or loss of mental faculties, such as memory loss, brain fatigue and inability to 'figure things out' may result. In my clinical experience, multiple sclerosis, muscular dystrophy, myasthenia gravis, Bell's palsy, cyclical headaches (including migraines), hardening of the arteries, diseases of the vital organs, extreme weight loss or weight gain, tinnitus, sleep imbalances, all indicate thyroid troubles. All addictions will tend to imbalance the thyroid gland when it is overwhelmed by the concentrated chemical compounds contained in the abused substance.

All types of growth, tumours and cancer will be registered by the thyroid gland. Many of the substances that the thyroid secretes and releases to other parts of the body will change when the body is degenerating in any way from disease. Tumours are the result of the thyroid, as well as all the other glands and organs, not being able to resolve their imbalance. Even mental illnesses have a manifestation as biochemical imbalances. Unresolved emotional traumas throw the body off balance, and finally produce toxins and waste. This chemical imbalance distorts the ability of the nervous system to respond normally. Traumas can be 'locked' into the body, and experiencing similar circumstances can bring them to the surface.

What expresses itself physically through symptoms is also expressed emotionally or psychologically in some way and follows patterns of 'repetition'. Unresolved pain, guilt and suffering in childhood, created by years of parental disapproval and disappointment for example, establish recurring patterns of response to similar situations, until this cycle of activity is resolved in some way. These emotional traumas give rise to imbalance in the body via the thyroid gland.

FOODS

When the thyroid appears in your questionnaire result, the following adjustments need to be made with your foods. Increase the Phase Three foods to strengthen and support the thyroid (see the Five Phase food chart, p. 170). Increase your intake of millet, sweet potato, yams, artichokes, yellow squash, parsnips, pumpkin or gourd-like squashes (acorn, butternut, spaghetti squash), sweet corn, apples, papaya and pineapple. Increase watercress, leeks, celery, rice, swedes, walnuts, cottage cheese, yoghurt, salmon, tuna, swordfish, cod, flounder, haddock, halibut, herring and plaice. Reduce or avoid ice cream, cheese (especially highly ripened soft cheese), eggs, cauliflower, cabbage, white potato and soybeans in any form.

SUPPLEMENTS

By far the most important supplements for the thyroid are the minerals. Take a **multimineral** 1–3 times a day (see *Resources*). When there is a sluggish metabolism due to low thyroid activity (hypo-thyroidism), supplement with iodine, which is easily available from sea vegetables. Nori, wakame, hijiki and arame are all excellent natural food sources of iodine. Eat pickled sea vegetables 3–4 times weekly. If you prefer to supplement iodine in tablet form, only take a maximum of 3 tablets of 0.225mg daily until you have had a thyroid blood analysis; and make the food changes in your diet (see above).

Calcium supplements are essential to balance over- and under-active thyroid glands. When chemotherapy or radio-therapy is used in treating cancer, the thyroid is bombarded in an attempt to further production of 'wild' cancer cells. Calcium protects the cell membrane where blood goes back and forth. It is the most vital mineral to counteract the effects of acidity. Take 500mg of calcium, 1–3 times daily as either aspartate, chelate or EAP form for acute or chronic conditions that affect the thyroid. Vitamin C as calcium or magnesium ascorbate cleanses the lymphatic system and the whole blood circulation. For acute conditions take 1,500mg 3 times a day. For chronic cases, take 1,000mg 1–3 times a day. Riboflavin and niacin (nicotinic acid) help support and stabilise iodine's metabolic activity – take 50–200mg daily (see *Resources*).

To stimulate the thyroid, homeopathic thyroid can be taken. Start with a 30c potency for acute conditions, taking 3 doses for 3 days. For chronic conditions of low thyroid activity take a single dose of 200c or 1m potency. Homeopathic Lycopodium (Club Moss) is the best remedy for overactivity of the thyroid, as it tends to slow down the rhythm of the gland. Take 6 c, 30c dosages for 3 days. Wait 1 month and if there is no improvement, try 3 more doses again for 3 consecutive days, as before. Otherwise, take the homeopathic remedies Reckeweg **R20** (for women) or **R19** (for men) as a support for the hypothalamus, pituitary and adrenal glands, and the testes or ovaries. If the condition is combined with acute or chronic trauma, take the above remedies combined with R55 for physical or emotional shocks or traumas. For weight-related thyroid disturbances (obesity), take R59. The Reckeweg remedies can be taken 3 times per day, 10–15 drops in half a glass of water.

Try using a positive thought for stimulating your thyroid.

'I am confident and fair with myself and others. I always do the right thing and think the best thoughts about myself and others.'

GROUP 11

The Veins, Arteries and Capillaries of the Circulatory System

PHASE TWO

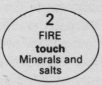

2
FIRE
touch
Minerals and
salts

For guidance on how to use the information in this section see p. 65.

When Group 11 appears in your questionnaire analysis, it indicates that an imbalance is affecting the veins and arteries throughout the body. All the vital organs receive blood to replenish nutrients. The blood bathes the tissues and removes waste matter for elimination from the body. Disturbances to the acid–alkaline balance of the body hamper the digestion, assimilation and utilisation of foods, and this means that undigested metabolites may endanger the vascular system. When blood does not move properly through the body, the veins and arteries may begin to bulge out or dilate, and this exerts pressure within the body. Just like a building designed to withstand certain pressure, so the veins and arteries, too, can only manage so much pressure from the blood as it moves through the system. Any weaknesses will break down under the pressure. This happens particularly at the intersections between arteries or veins, where it can produce varicose veins, haemorrhoids, calcium build-up, headaches, migraines or haemorrhages. Changes in the pressure of the flow from or into the heart may be due to internal or external factors.

Environmental pollutants and toxic waste alter the whole life cycle in nature and contribute to changes in the natural barometric pressures that produce our weather. These pressures affect blood flow and can also be responsible for changes of mood. Too many concentrated proteins, fats and carbohydrates, which are not digested, remain embedded and harden in the veins and arteries. Once this pattern is established, symptoms may manifest in a number of ways depending on individual and family weaknesses, damaging the vascular flow throughout the body. Left untreated this can lead to forms of heart disease. Physical blockages can create emotional blockages, represented by resentments towards oneself and others. Blockages in the veins and arteries can affect the way one feels in general: the individual may lose a sense of 'lightness', playfulness and no longer enjoy the game of life. Such people feel 'heavy' and it becomes a laborious chore just to move around in daily life. People with arterial blockage and vascular stagnation find great difficulty in making and keeping their own personal commandments (agreements with themselves) to action, and often procrastinate when it comes to giving themselves the joyful fruits of the body, mind and spirit.

FOODS

In conditions affecting the veins and arteries, increase the Phase One vegetables, grains, beans, fish, nuts, dairy products (see the Five Phase food chart, p. 170). In particular eat more corn, asparagus, chicory, endive, escarole, okra (lady's finger), green onions, artichoke, broccoli, carrots, lettuces (especially cos, but not iceberg), apricots, sharon fruit, raspberries, strawberries, sunflower seeds and prawns. Avoid eggs, all shellfish, mushrooms, watermelon, blackberry, blueberry, cranberry, kidney beans, pinto beans, black beans. Avoid Phase Five foods, especially the grains, beans, meats, nuts and seeds.

SUPPLEMENTS

The most important supplement, for both its cleansing and building properties, is vitamin C in the form of **calcium or magnesium ascorbate**. In acute conditions take 500–1,000mg every 4–6 hours, especially for haemorrhaging, painful varicose veins and headaches. For chronic problems take 1,000–2,000mg 3 times a day. **Bioflavonoids**, a component of vitamin C, strengthen the veins and arteries including the capillaries. Take 1,000–2,000mg daily. Vitamin B3 (niacin) helps cleanse and clear debris from the veins and arteries by re-stimulating incomplete energy cycles, igniting the food as fuel to be consumed by the 'fire' properties that niacin contains. For acute problems take 100–300mg, 3–6 times a day. For chronic vascular congestion take 500–1,000mg 3 times a day. Make sure that you always take vitamin C and calcium or magnesium to buffer the effects of niacin. Rutin, another component of the vitamin C complex, is derived from the grain buckwheat. It strengthens the walls of the arteries, veins and capillaries. Take 100–300mg twice daily. Alternatively take the homeopathic remedy Reckeweg R42 for varicose veins or eczema. In acute cases take 10 drops 3 times a day; in chronic cases 20–30 drops once a day before bed. General inflammation and cramps in the lower extremities in chronic cases take 10–15 drops of Reckeweg R63 3 times a day, half an hour before meals. In chronic cases a drop of R1 3 times a day should be taken.

Try using a positive thought for strengthening the circulatory system.

'I am flowing and moving with my life lovingly.'

GROUP 12

The Brain and the Central Nervous System

PHASES TWO AND THREE

2	3
FIRE	**EARTH**
touch	**taste**
Minerals and salts	Sugars and carbohydrates

For guidance on how to use the information in this section see p. 65.

When Group 12 appears in your questionnaire analysis, it indicates that your stress levels are high, creating nervousness and problems with the nervous system. As technology, information, and the pace of modern urban living speeds up, we all run the risk that we will lose sight of the basic simplicity of life. Time becomes an enemy of the changing world we live in. When life gets too complicated, we lose our ability to see ourselves clearly, and to be truthful about our relationships with the people, places and things in our lives. Our ability to sort out the meaning of our 'life story' from beginning to end becomes blocked by physical, emotional and spiritual trauma. This in turn places pressure on the healthy interrelationship of body, mind and spirit.

All events in our lives are measured in time. Time is recorded on calendars, which are our way of keeping track of our experiences. Our understanding of the physical universe depends on our concept of time. In medieval days, time was based in part on the radiation of silver. Today, as the dictionary describes, a second is based on the period of radiation corresponding to the transition between 2 hyperfine levels of a ground-state ceasium-133 atom. Time is, in 1 sense, imposed upon us; many of us feel there is not enough of it! Constant stress on time and the urgency to complete tasks excites the nervous system. This, combined with the environmental pressures on the body, mind and spirit makes the brain feel overwhelmed and nervous.

Residual physical and emotional stress at night prevents the mind from slowing enough to rest and sleep. The body becomes so exhausted that the mind cannot shut off, which is 1 of the underlying conditions that produces insomnia. The nature of physical energy is that if 1 area or zone of the body is blocked by nerve congestion, the body will compensate in another area in an attempt to restore neutrality and equilibrium. This conditioning can produce twitches, tics, incoherent electrical patterns in the 'sleep centres' of the brain and a host of other imbalances that prevent the brain from distinguishing reality from unreality.

The nervous system regulates the movement of electrical impulses through the nerve pathways to every nerve sheath in the body. The brain and the nervous system conduct messages about every person, place or object in the environment. These messages are translated into information that reaches all the gland and organ structures (which can be thought of as sub-brains, and chemical command centres). We need to simplify our daily existence and create a more tranquil environment for the nervous system. We also need to eat healthy balanced foods, exercise to keep the body supple and commune with the beauty in nature.

FOODS
The single most important factor in considering how best to support the nervous system is to avoid eating too many 'condensed' foods, which include flesh foods, cheese and all dairy products, alcohol, sugars, coffee, teas, shellfish and salt. Over-stimulating the nervous system creates too much 'current' through the nerves. Sedating the nervous system creates too little. Either too much or too little 'current' creates a sugar imbalance. This produces a toxic state of

affairs in the biochemistry of the body, and poisons the brain and
entire network of nerves that feed information to all the tissues,
glands and organs. In chemical terms, the 'voltage' passing
through foods is fats, proteins, carbohydrates, and (most
importantly) sugars which fuel all the activity that animates the
body. Taking too much of any 1 category of foods will distort the
experience of the nervous system. Too much of anything, as
already discussed, produces an increased positive charge, and
therefore pressure and pain from acidity. Too little causes a
negative charge, which produces alkalinity. This in turn gives
rise to mental sensations, such as feeling 'spaced out'. For
disturbances to the nervous system, increase Phase Two and
Phase Three foods with reference to the Five Phase food chart
on p. 170. Focus especially on the vegetables from Phase Two
and Phase Three. Vegetables are the most balancing foods for
the nervous system because they supply minerals that are often
lacking when the nerves are under stress. Avoid all pulses; they
will disturb the digestion and block the absorption of other
nutrients. Reduce wheat, oats, rye, barley, peppers, mushrooms, oranges, grapefruit, brazil nuts, cashews, butter,
cream, sour cream, eggs. Avoid all sour foods, pickles, vinegar,
sauerkraut, coffee, tea, tobacco, salt and all foods containing
yeast.

SUPPLEMENTS

Take a **B-complex** supplement (see *Resources*). In acute
cases, 25–75mg 1–3 times a day; for chronic conditions,
50–75mg once a day. This supports and rebuilds the myelin
sheath – the nerve coating. For mineral supplementation take
calcium EAP, in acute cases, 500–1,000mg 2–3 times a day; for
chronic conditions, 500–1,500mg 1–2 times a day. Magnesium
EAP should also be taken. In acute cases 250–500mg 2–4 times
a day; for chronic conditions, 500–750mg 1–2 times a day.

The Reckeweg homeopathic remedies to look for are R14,
which are nerve and sleep drops to be taken with the above
supplements. R14 helps to reduce the physical and emotional

pressure on the nervous system. In acute cases take 10 drops every 3–4 hours; for chronic conditions, take 15 drops upon rising and before sleep. **Vita-C-15** (see *Resources*) is a tonic for all acute and chronic stress on the nerves and muscles that is causing tension, nervousness and anxiety. For acute cases take 1 teaspoon every 4–6 hours; in chronic conditions, especially for sleep, 1 teaspoon after breakfast and lunch, and 1 tablespoon before bed.

Try using a positive thought for stimulating your nervous system.

'I am always in perfect time and space for my life. I am simple, whole and complete.'

GROUP 13

The Adrenal Glands and the Energy System

PHASE FIVE

(
5
WATER
hearing
Water
)

For guidance on how to use the information in this section see p. 65.

The adrenal glands are the 'spark plugs' of the body. They release substances that ignite the whole energy conversion cycle. As food breaks down into energy through metabolism the adrenals coordinate and help to regulate the work of the pancreas and liver. In fact, the adrenal glands, pancreas and liver make the major gland/organ energy triad in the body. The adrenal glands increase and decrease the body's capacity for energy and significantly affect the way the body, mind and spirit ascend to higher levels of development and personal wisdom, or descend into physically limited, ego-bound patterns that repeat themselves and limit personal growth and development. The chemistry of the adrenal glands produces the 'fight or flight' reaction and controls the physical instinct to be under stress and 'win'. When the adrenal functions are low, there will be a physical and emotional low, and the body and mind will not be able to cope with pressure. The individual will lose the battle with the environment, as the environmental pollutants rob energy from the body and disturb the regulation of the body chemistry.

For example, when the adrenals are low, stress can produce low blood sugar. Low blood sugar affects 1 out of 3 people today living in an urban environment. Orthodox medicine is not geared up to respond to marginal problems of low blood sugar. Without sensitive tests for low blood sugar, patients will not be properly diagnosed as having adrenal exhaustion until the syndrome is established. Sugar cravings, exhaustion, concentration problems, excessive worry, feeling drained of energy between 2 p.m. and 6 p.m., sleep troubles, mental highs and lows (especially at night), are some of the major symptoms of adrenal exhaustion.

Fifty per cent of people suffering from depression have depressed adrenal activity. When depression affects the body, mind and spirit, day-to-day difficulties make the individual feel ashamed and humiliated, lacking self-esteem, unable to cope and to feel proud. Such adrenal lows undermine the courage and confidence to live life to the full.

The physical–biochemical condition and the emotional imbalance go hand in hand. There is no separation between the physical and emotional, the biochemical and mental! They are 2 sides of the same coin.

When the adrenal glands are low for an extended period of time, the body may try to recreate a balance by secreting extra insulin and adrenalin. Diabetes may result from chronic excesses of these chemicals. Diabetes comes about when the body loses its ability to absorb, manufacture, distribute and dispose of the sugar (glucose) properly. The system is flooded with glucose and it 'burns' up specific areas of the body because of its high concentration. This causes excessive acidity (diabetic acidosis) which produces swelling, pain and inflammation, and may lead to disturbances in the optic centre because of increased pressure on the eyes and brain centres.

Highs or lows of sugar in the metabolism will disrupt the entire metabolic pathway of fats, proteins and carbohydrates. This is why so many diabetics gain weight; they are not able to make energy, use the energy and eliminate waste. Instead they store the incomplete energy as fat.

FOODS

The remedy for high or low sugar conditions is to balance the food by stabilising the utilisation of carbohydrates. In either case, a careful regime of the correct complex carbohydrates, plus supplementation, will almost always stabilise the imbalanced metabolism of a diabetic. Follow strictly the 2 diets given in Chapter Four. Eat a carbohydrate breakfast, protein lunch and carbohydrate–protein dinner. As a rule increase Phase Four and Phase Five foods, referring to the Five Phase food chart on p. 170.

Snacks between meals are essential to improve the sugar balance. Between breakfast and lunch, focus on your carbohydrate intake: crispbreads, oatcakes, rice cakes with a small amount of honey or preserve containing only natural fruit sugar. Or choose some cooked grain: about 100g of rice or millet. Fresh vegetable juices are excellent because of their 'live enzyme' content, which is vital for re-establishing stable energy patterns. Disturbances of the adrenal glands that affect the blood sugar always affect enzyme levels as well. To make a juice to improve digestion, take 2 carrots, 2 stalks of celery, half a bunch of medium size parsley, half a bunch of watercress and 1 medium size raw beet, peeled. Put this through a juicer and add a good squeeze of lemon juice. Drink the concoction slowly, allowing the juice to mix well with the saliva. According to the work of Dr Norman Walker, juices can work miracles in restoring body chemistry to balance.

Between lunch and dinner eat some protein; combine 7–14 almonds, 50g sunflower seeds, 50g pumpkin seeds, 100–150g live yoghurt and the same quantity of cottage cheese. Have a small amount of carbohydrate with this protein between lunch and dinner, such as crackers, crispbreads, oatcakes, brown toast or a jacket potato.

SUPPLEMENTS

Unequivocally the most important vitamin for stress is **pantothenic acid**, probably the single most important extra nutrient that we need. For acute tiredness, fatigue or lethargy, take 500–1,000mg with breakfast and lunch. Do not take it at night because it may tend to stimulate the brain centres and inhibit sleep. As a general rule, stop taking the supplement at 7 p.m. For pain or inflammation related to arthritis or other bone troubles, take 2,000–4,000mg every 3–4 hours. For chronic tiredness take 1,000–1,500mg after breakfast and lunch, and again 2 hours after lunch.

From the homeopathic collection, choose R86, which is designed to work on blood sugar troubles. In acute cases, take 10 drops every 2–3 hours; for chronic conditions, 15 drops in half a glass of water, 3 times a day. For diagnosed diabetes take R40. In acute cases when the blood sugar is particularly high take 10 drops every 4 hours. For chronic diabetes take 10 drops 3 times a day.

Try using a positive thought for stimulating your adrenal glands.

'I am courageous with my physical, emotional and spiritual energy now and forever.'

The Mind–Body Connection

ALL FIVE PHASES

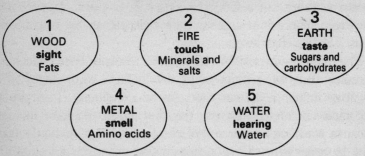

For guidance on how to use the information in this section see p. 65.

In our world today the mind is being contaminated by many different persons, places and things. The mind analyses and evaluates everything in the environment and has a 'collective', unconscious memory for all the past history and experiences that have taken place since the beginning of recorded time. Carl Jung formulated this hypothesis in the early part of this century before humanity faced the horrors of World War Two and the threat of fascism. Fascism represents the major degeneration of thought in our age. Episodes in our past, such as the holocaust, represent the furthest that the mind has moved from truth and goodness, wisdom and love.

Since World War Two and the rise of technology, the speed at which we can influence people through propaganda and the press has meant that we have succumbed to a level of information poisoning that has never existed before. Powerful images, symbols, colour and sound have the ability to overpower the individual. The result of such superficial manipulation is that the individual becomes a victim controlled. The only way to be able to resist such powers is for the individual to be in touch with his or her own feelings, and to be able to give 'real' meaning to life and living. Otherwise, misleading and often dangerous images are stored in the memory and can be activated under conditions of pressure and stress. The mind is designed to use its memory banks of stored information from the past in order to deal with the present. Many people who are not sufficiently conscious of their own feelings, however, suppress or repress their feelings, unable to come to grips with their past experiences.

The mind needs positive affirmations to experience peace and serenity. But what most of us are being exposed to has a negative influence on our thoughts and feelings. Therefore it becomes useful to feed the mind beautiful, positive images because we need a point and place of equilibrium and a point of rest in order to achieve balance. Without such a route for regaining equilibrium, people become addicted to habits or drugs in order to escape from the difficulties of their day-to-day experience, even if it is just a momentary escape from the pain. No drug is completely free from side effects. The history of drugs is the history of humans wanting to be free of pain and suffering. Drugs have the opposite effect to foods. Instead of nourishing and feeding the cells they super-charge the individual to extreme states of pressure, giving rise to pains and sensations caused by excess states of acidity or alkalinity.

Nourishing the mind is not separate from nourishing the body. The foods that we eat, the substances that we ingest, the air that we breathe, are all part and parcel of the overall nourishment for the body, mind and spirit. Our society today is being poisoned in many ways and on many levels. This violence against ourselves endangers the survival of the species. Only by using our mind for the highest good can we overcome the destruction of the last hundred years. The challenge has to be faced at the level of the individual, learning to listen to the self, and not trying to follow belief systems that cannot keep up with the pace of change. If we can use our minds for truth, wisdom, love, understanding, compassion and cooperation, then we can begin the long process of discovery that we are all on.

FOODS

Eat all foods moderately, focusing on a balanced diet that takes in foods from all the Phases (see the Five Phase food chart on p. 170). If Group 14 appears as the first number (box A) in your questionnaire analysis, set up your nourishment cycle based on your second number (box B) in your report by turning to that group number and following the dietary advice given there.

If Group 14 appears as your second number (box B), then set up your Five Phase nourishment cycle based on the first number group, by turning to the section for that group and following the dietary advice.

In any case avoid sugar, tea, coffee and red meat (once to twice a week maximum). Reduce dairy products, especially cheese, milk, cream and butter. Avoid pork products such as luncheon meats, ham and sausages, and also cooked oils and tobacco products.

SUPPLEMENTS

Take 2 capsules of a **multivitamin** (see *Resources*) twice a day in acute cases, once a day for chronic problems. Use multiminerals as well (see *Resources*); in acute cases 1 capsule 3 times a day, for chronic problems, 2 capsules with lunch or dinner. Take 1 capsule of NT188 at breakfast and dinner.

From the homeopathic remedies, choose R14 for nervousness, tension, anxiety or panic. In acute cases take 1 teaspoon every 3–4 hours; for chronic problems 1 teaspoon 3 times a day and an extra dose before bed. Vit-A-C-15 is a tonic to calm the mind and relax the nervous system. In acute cases take 1 teaspoon every 4–6 hours; for chronic problems, 1 teaspoon 3 times a day and an extra dose 1 hour before bed.

Try using a positive thought for stimulating the mind.

'I am analysing and comprehending my life so I get what I really want.'

The Sensory Mechanism (Sight, Touch, Taste, Smell and Hearing)

ALL FIVE PHASES

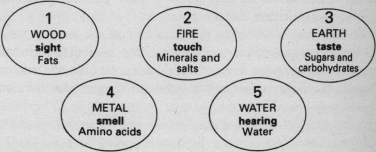

For guidance on how to use the information in this section see p. 65.

Through the senses the human being receives, tracks and records the impact of all persons, places and things. We respond to the threats that all other life forms exert over us. Historically, the body has been prepared to 'eat or be eaten'. This has been our biological imperative. We test our safety by measuring the size, mass and strength of all competitors, and we do this through a genetically programmed response.

Our evaluation of the environment through our sensory mechanism demands that we pay attention as we move through time and space, through the 'urban jungle'. Because of the fast-moving nature of our environment, our senses are constantly being overwhelmed as well as violated by the various forms of pollution: sound pollution, visual pollution, taste pollution, olfactory (smell) pollution, touch pollution and speech pollution. The body's solution to this is to become 'unconscious' and 'turn off'. In this condition it becomes more and more difficult for the individual to be in control of him or herself. The challenge assumes great proportions – to survive and develop as a whole and complete human being or to be slowly worn down by an increasingly stressful environment. We must discover a whole new way of being adaptable to the circumstances, which begins with simply accepting 'what is'. The only alternative is to revolt and rest, denying 'what is' and working constantly in the hope of making it 'go away'.

From the point of view of the individual, it is wiser perhaps to begin by accepting the existence of such 'poisons', and once having accepted that, to take a view on what to do about it. Any denial of 'what is' leads the individual into an unconscious state, no longer in a position to be in control. This level of denial of our surroundings applies to our eating habits, too. Every time we bypass the effort necessary to put food on the table by using convenience foods or 'take-aways', something in us becomes unconscious. We lose our connection with the world around us and miss out on the creative process of making beautiful food for our body, mind and spirit.

Given that the first step towards self-realisation is acceptance of 'what is', THE FELT FORMULA accepts also the realistic proposition of 'balancing your poisons'. This means to discover a day-to-day strategy for living, and a means towards moderation. This begins with losing your fear of any food, any person, place or thing and rediscovering that, even under extreme conditions, all things continue to work. Keep an open mind and body so that you can discover for yourself how life works. In this way we can share the best with ourselves and each other, and not be inhibited by the environment with all its threats!

In conclusion, we must re-educate our senses and extend them to their full potential by coping with this modern challenge. We have much untapped human mind- will-, and brain-power. The senses, through the ears, nose, skin, eyes and tongue give us our potential to both express and receive all forms of natural beauty. For it is beauty that under even the most extreme conditions feeds the human spirit and soul.

FOOD

When Group 15 appears in your questionnaire analysis as the first or second number it indicates either acute or chronic toxicity. Often this condition is accompanied by extreme weight gain or loss, poor skin and low energy levels. The most important adjustment is to cut out all junk foods, processed foods, foods with additives and preservatives, white flour, white sugar, cakes, candies, biscuits, fizzy drinks and red meat for at least a couple of months. Increasing the foods that are high in enzymes will detoxify the system and clean up the bloodstream. Foods that are particularly suitable are watercress, parsley, rocket, mustard and cress, radiccio, escarole, endive, chicory and lettuces (red and green). Follow the proportions given in the two diets on p. 41, using the carbohydrate and protein menus alternately.

SUPPLEMENTS

Take spirulina; in acute cases, 3 tablets 4–6 times daily, for chronic conditions 4 tablets twice daily. Also take enzymes (see Digest-acid, in *Resources*); in acute cases, 1 capsule after breakfast, lunch and dinner. For chronic conditions, 2 tablets after lunch and dinner. Take vitamin C as calcium or magnesium ascorbate. In acute cases, 1,500mg, 3–4 times a day; for chronic conditions, 1,000–2,000mg 1–2 times a day.

From the homeopathic remedies use **R26**, the draining and stimulating drops. In acute cases, 10 drops 4 times a day; for chronic conditions, 15 drops twice a day, upon rising and before bed. Also use **R60**, the blood purifier, in acute cases 10 drops 4 times a day, for chronic conditions 15 drops twice a day, upon rising and before bed.

Try using a positive thought for stimulating the mind.

'I am expressing thoughts clearly and paying the result I create.'

The Kidneys, Bladder, Urethra and Prostate

PHASE FIVE

5
WATER
hearing
Water

For guidance on how to use the information in this section see p.
65.

When Group 16 appears as the first or second number in your
questionnaire analysis it means that your body is not purifying
your blood properly or efficiently, which is causing problems
with the filtration system of the body. A large portion of the
body's wastes and poisons are eliminated through the kidneys.
By purifying the blood and eliminating poisons, the kidneys
work by distinguishing the 'life' from the 'death' principles within
the body. Blood and waste is separated and the purified blood
returns to the heart to be circulated throughout the body. In
this way the heart and kidneys have a very close relationship.
Disturbances to the kidney can produce Addison's disease,
Bright's disease, cystitis, urethritis and painful swelling and
inflammation of the bladder, causing frequency of urination. In
men this problem can lead to a swelling of the prostate. All
kidney problems begin with an acid–alkaline imbalance (see p.
44). Severe imbalances affecting the kidneys and the bladder
cause contractions of the ducts of the kidneys (nephrons),
which control the flow of urine out of the body, so that too much
or too little urine leaves the body. When the refuse of the body
is not eliminated properly the body can be overrun with waste
and toxic poisons. If the kidneys are unable to purify the waste,

calcium and other by-products may begin to be deposited in the kidneys and other vital organs. This may lead to arterial sclerosis, or a hardening or thickening of the organs, tissues, or vessels arising from inflammation, degeneration and deposits of fatty plaques.

Even in the Bible, where the foundations of modern medicine can be found, it says 'the Lord searches and tries the reins (kidneys) and heart . . .' The reins of the body (or kidneys) are referred to in the Psalms and in Jeremiah. The condition of kidneys reflects the purity of the being.

According to Oriental medicine, kidney troubles produce symptoms affecting the ears and hearing. The individual will also crave salty foods. She or he will suffer from cold extremities (hands and feet), especially at night. Early hair loss may be another symptom. Any stress can produce shakiness and the person may appear a bit unsteady or quivery and the body and voice may tremble. Fear and panic attacks are the emotional manifestation of kidney problems. The sense of individual emotional autonomy and of will and personal power may be low.

FOODS
The most important dietary change is to reduce all acid-forming foods: bread, potatoes, tomatoes, mushrooms, oranges, grapefruit, spinach, peppers, peanuts, cashews, pistachios, brazil nuts, cream, cheese, sour cream, milk, white flour, white sugar, cakes, biscuits, candies, chocolate, alcohol, shellfish, aubergine, cauliflower, cabbage, brussel sprouts. All these foods tend to increase levels of albumen, a protein by-product. When proteins are not assimilated they come through the digestive system and may promote congestion in the kidneys.

Foods to increase are: generally all leafy green vegetables, and especially broccoli, watercress, savoy cabbage, green peas, parsley, courgettes, lettuces, celery, chinese cabbage, beetroot, yams, sweet potato, acorn squash, butternut squash, spaghetti squash. The grains to increase are millet and buckwheat. Avoid pulses in general, as well as wheat and oats.

SUPPLEMENTS
For women:
Take a multivitamin (see *Resources*) with breakfast and lunch
and 1 capsule of each of Ligazyme, Acidophilus and the herb
Uva ursi at breakfast, lunch and dinner. For cystitis take 2
tablets of Cantharis 6 upon rising for 6 days.

The homeopathic remedy R1 will help inflammation. In acute
cases take 10 drops every 3–4 hours; in chronic cases 10 drops
should be taken 3 times a day. Also you should take **R18**, 10
drops every 3–4 hours if you have an acute problem; 10 drops 3
times a day if your problem is chronic.
For men:
For prostate and bladder troubles take either the herb Saw
Palmetto, 1 capsule at breakfast and lunch or the homeopathic
remedy Sabal Serrulata, 2 tablets upon rising for 6 days. For
inflammation you should take Reckeweg R1 in the same dosage
as set out for women above and also the same dosage of **R25**.

Try using a positive thought for stimulating the kidneys.

'I am purifying my body, mind and spirit, making it fit and
balanced.'

The Male–Female Hormone Balance and the Endocrine System

AL FIVE PHASES

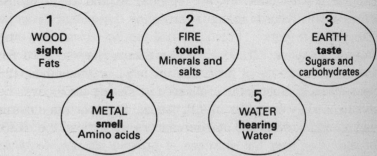

For guidance on how to use the information in this section see p. 65.

The endocrine hormones are secretions from a variety of glands and organs that help to restore equilibrium whenever the body goes to chemical and emotional extremes due to stress of any sort. The glands and organs that create the circuit of the endocrine system are: the adrenals, thymus, hypothalamus, pancreas, testes/ovaries, thyroid, pituitary and parathyroid. Every diagnosable disease involves the hormones in some way. Whenever the body and mind experience loss of energy ('hypo'conditions), or 'hyper' conditions involving excess, the hormones lose their equilibrium. At any point in time both 'excess' and 'lack' may be present in the body to some degree. The excessive state represents acute types of conditions; the lacking state produces sensations or ailments of a chronic sort.

The hormones coordinate with the entire biochemistry of the body in order to live as long as possible in the most comfortable fashion, from the biochemical point of view. The hormones restore, rebalance, equalise and conserve all the vital substances of the body in all their forms. Given the state of the environment, it is a tall order for the hormones to be able to perform the job for which nature designed them. The hormones are somewhat like a group of people running around a room in chaos because the lights have been turned off and everyone and everything is being knocked over!

Many of the complaints that affect women in particular today, can be traced back (in my opinion) to the effect of the environment disturbing and interrupting the genetic programming for procreation. Pre-menstrual tension, thrush and other vaginal disorders, PID (Pelvic Inflammatory Disease), endometriosis, the effects of birth control pills, oestrogen therapy, miscarriages, amenorrhea (absence of menstruation), cystitis, dysmenorrhea (irregular menstruation), osteoporosis, arthritis and breast, cervical and uterine cancers are some of the results of this. For men the increase of prostate cancer, testicular cancer and male breast cancer can to a certain degree be traced back to the low levels of poisoning present in our environment. Our biochemistry was not designed to be exposed to such subtle forms of energy and thus our hormones cannot easily adapt to the normal conditions of living. The resulting chemical stress on the endocrine system speeds up the ageing process. Eating poor quality foods compounds the problems and sets the stage for many disorders.

Marginal ill health affects many people; one of the major problems is not having enough energy or having poor stamina, which prevents the individual from experiencing a sense of harmony physically, emotionally and spiritually. The results may be a mild symptom, mood swings or fluid problems, or severe symptoms such as the distorted, perverted experiences and complete personality changes that some women experience when going through the menopause. In either case the hormones regulate so many functions in the body that when they are disturbed it affects the entire sensory mechanism. This may exaggerate experiences one way or the other, making things seem too big or too small. Harmony, balance and a sense of well-being are thwarted.

FOODS

A balanced diet is more important for hormonal conditions than any others. Hormonal imbalances often make people go to extremes in their eating patterns. Sugar, chocolate, breads and starches are some of the foods that people with hormonal problems characteristically crave. When these foods are taken to excess they exaggerate the imbalance and mask the original condition. The 2 recommended diets (see p. 41), used in the sequence breakfast–carbohydrate, lunch–protein, dinner–carbohydrate, will help restore a balance. If there are energy problems, eat snacks between meals to help maintain balance. Refer to the snack designs on p. 41.

SUPPLEMENTS

Taking a good **multivitamin** (see *Resources*) is essential to support all the endocrine system and the hormonal balance. For acute problems take 1 capsule or tablet twice a day; for chronic troubles take a multivitamin 3 times a day. Also vital to hormone balance are the unsaturated fatty acids. GLA is a very important fatty acid (see *Resources*); take 500–1,500mg 1–3 times a day. For extra support, women can take both angelica (obtainable as the Chinese **Dong Quai**), and agnus castus 1–3 times a day. Men should take **Ginseng**, 500mg 1–3 times a day along with 400–1,000i.u. of vitamin E, (dry succinate or d-alpha tocopherol form).

For period problems the addition of vitamin B6 is helpful. Take it as Pyridoxyl-5-Phosphate, 50–150mg daily. Pantothenic acid (vitamin B5) can be taken 1–3 times a day, 500–1,500mg. For severe energy loss, take the amino acid tyrosine, which supports the adrenal glands and the entire endocrine hormonal balance; 500–1,000mg between meals will help restore lost energy.

Homeopathic remedy R19 for men supports the hormones; take 10–15 drops 1–3 times a day. For women, use R20, 10–15 drops 1–3 times a day in half a glass of water.

Try using a positive thought for stimulating the endocrine system.

'I am conserving, preserving and deserving my physical, emotional and spiritual energy reserves.'

GROUP 19

The Skin and the Excretory System

PHASE FOUR

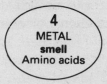

4
METAL
smell
Amino acids

For guidance on how to use the information in this section see p. 65.

The skin is one of the major links to the heart and circulatory system. It is connected to the walls of the arteries and hence to the whole of the circulation and the glands and organs.

The skin eliminates waste through exhalations of dead matter through the pores. Many substances are also absorbed by the skin. This makes it one of the first areas of the body to react to any threat from outside. If there is a real danger, the hairs on the skin may stand up and feel sensitive and prickly. This is a sign for the rest of the body to be aware, and to be on guard. There is nothing that can override these automatic warnings for the individual.

The condition of the skin reveals much about the condition of the whole body. The particular location of skin problems can indicate the origin of the problem, by their position relative to specific acupuncture points and meridians, or 'energy pathways'. Each meridian is connected to a specific internal location. A skilful diagnostic specialist can see where the problems are coming from and how the body is attempting to push out poisons and toxins. Skin problems such as eczema, psoriasis, seborrhoea and dermatitis are in a large part due to the build up of waste that is not being properly eliminated. Like chinks in armour the skin cracks, abrasions, dryness, flaking and chafing are also signs of the imbalances from within. This waste build up pushes the body chemistry to extreme acidity. The internal acidity of the body determines how the skin is faring. This means that cosmetic attempts to change the acidity of the skin are unlikely to have much effect.

The oils and fats that lubricate the body and help regulate fatty acid metabolism are vital for healthy skin and hair.

The characteristic emotional changes that are associated with the skin being out of balance are a loss of dynamism, and possibly boredom, which is suppressed anger. The individual may feel like a victim of circumstance, and completely out of control with no real direction or purpose in life. This is to do with unconscious hurts, wounds and pains from life before the age of 6 which have become patterned in the body. Many types of birth traumas or early sexual abuse may become visible in skin troubles. I have seen many cases of this and am aware of the protestations from the individual who feels sure that there are no buried emotional problems. It is character-istic for skin troubles to be related to unconscious thoughts that are suppressed and repressed deep within. When the condition is treated nutritionally and the emotions that are buried or hidden are talked about, the skin starts to ooze. This indicates that the suppressed emotions are starting to flow once again. Often the skin clears up permanently within a short while as long as the individual is willing to face their own inner 'story'.

Many people with skin problems tend to exacerbate them by eating the wrong foods. They crave and desire the very foods that make their condition worse and use skin preparations to mask their condition which inflame the skin more. There is nothing worse for the body and mind than the denial of 'what is'. Diet and nutrition can help clear the skin, but at the same time awareness of the feelings of the body, mind and spirit is equally important. The one without the other will not promote enduring optimal health.

FOODS

When there are skin disturbances the body needs to cut out toxins and anything other than wholefoods. Avoid the following foods for 30–45 days: breads, cheese, milk, tomatoes, spinach, mushrooms, peppers, white flour, white sugars, diet sodas and sugary drinks, oranges, grapefruit, tea, coffee, wheat, oats, peanuts, cashews, alcohol, pork products, smoked meats, shellfish, salt, all processed foods, packaged foods and preservative-ridden foods. In short follow a wholefood diet with fresh foods that are unadulterated.

Breakfast: whole grain cereals – cooked millet or cooked rice, or muesli. Use yoghurt or apple, grape or cranberry juice to moisten the cereal. Follow this with eggs and crackers, choosing from crispbreads, oatcakes or ricecakes with a little butter or jam without added sugar.

Lunch: green salad (all leafy green lettuces, parsley, watercress, mustard and cress, radiccio, endive, escarole or chicory) and protein: tuna, salmon (tinned), turkey breast, chicken breast, eggs, pilchards or sardines. Alternatively: rice (basmati or brown), jacket potato, sweet potato, yams, pasta (good semolina Italian pasta).

SUPPLEMENTS

The most important vitamin supplement is a well-balanced **multivitamin** (see *Resources*) that will be absorbed easily into the system. For acute skin problems take a multivitamin once or twice daily, for chronic problems take a multivitamin 1–3 times daily. Mega doses are unnecessary when the emphasis is put on eating properly. **Echinacea** will also have beneficial effects: take 15 drops 3 times a day. Liquid Vitamin A is very helpful for the skin. For acute problems take 10,000i.u. (1 drop) 3 times a day, for chronic conditions take 20,000i.u. (2 drops) twice a day. Also take zinc, 25mg 3 times a day for acute conditions; 50mg 3 times a day for chronic conditions.

From the homeopathic remedies use **R60**, the blood purifying drops. In acute cases, take 10–15 drops twice daily, for chronic conditions take 30 drops once a day before bed. The R93 immune fortifying drops are a useful addition. In acute cases take 15 drops upon rising and before bed; for chronic problems, 30 drops before bed.

Try using a positive thought for stimulating the skin.

'I am winning and succeeding physically, emotionally and spiritually.'

GROUP 20

The Pancreas and the Energy System

PHASE THREE

```
      3
    EARTH
    taste
   Sugars and
  carbohydrates
```

For guidance on how to use the information in this section see p. 65.

The major function of the pancreas is the regulation and distribution of insulin and the enzymes that are necessary for the digestion of starches, fats and proteins. The pancreas works via the liver and the adrenal glands to control the energy supply. It helps to convert carbohydrates into simple sugar, ready for intestinal absorption and utilisation. The pancreas gives the body the qualities of sweetness, empathy and sympathy expressed by the individual.

'The pancreas joins in the work of the spleen by setting aside from the current of thought . . . all that is unnecessarily acrimonious and severe, reserving this for kindliness, and the sense of superior merit and virtue, which need some rebuke, and sending forward sympathetic and friendly feelings which enter heartily, without censoriousness, into good uses.'(John Worcester, ibid.)

When there are imbalances in the pancreas the joy, laughter and lightness of the body are suppressed. Problems with the pancreas often manifest as blood sugar problems. This type of energy imbalance is often acute and severe, producing mood swings and an 'up and down' energy rhythm. Diabetes is the major disturbance to the sugar metabolism, the result of imbalances in the pancreas and, therefore, in the utilisation of carbohydrates.

Excess acidity in the body pulls sugar into the bloodstream supply. Acidity promotes the build up of chemical barriers, which prevents the proper digestion, absorption, assimilation and utilisation of food. Incomplete utilisation of starches prevents the body from feeling good or satisfied.

One of the signs of pancreatic and blood sugar problems is a bad taste in the mouth that causes bad breath. Pancreatic cancer is by far the most fatal type of cancer because of the role of the pancreas in the entire energy system.

A craving for sweets is one of the signs of pancreatic insufficiency. It suggests that the quality and quantity of carbohydrate being consumed is not right for the individual. Many people eat too much white sugar, white flour, cakes, candies, biscuits and ice cream – all the foods that are concentrated with the quick-acting sugars which supply no other nutrition. This and the acidity in the environment affect energy production. There will be a tendency for the individual to feel numerous unexplainable sensations such as over-reaction to stress, low stamina, feelings of paranoia and a general congestion in the head, throat and sinuses.

FOOD

When Group 20 appears as the first number (box A) in your questionnaire analysis it means that there are acute problems with the quality and endurance of your energy, both physically and emotionally, and especially during the daytime. This is a sign that your diet needs radical adjustment and you need to pay a great deal more attention to your body to prevent exhaustion. The easiest and most efficient plan of action is to follow the meal and diets on p. 39. Avoid the following foods: white flour products, white sugar, cakes, candies, biscuits, all refined sugar and starch products, packaged foods with preservatives.

Reduce your fruit consumption, particularly oranges and grape-fruits; reduce your intake of coffee, tea, fizzy drinks, diet sodas, alcohol, tobacco. Increase your consumption of green leafy vegetables and eat more broccoli, green beans, green peas, courgettes, parsley, asparagus, brussel sprouts, chicory, endive, escarole, okra (lady's fingers), jerusalem artichokes, greens, chard, parsnips, pumpkins and any gourd-like squashes – acorn, butternut and spaghetti squash and sweet corn. Reduce the Phase One grains, beans, nuts, seeds, dairy products, fish and meats. Avoid excessive quantities of oils or fats, pickles, vinegar or yeasted foods, such as Marmite and Vegemite.

SUPPLEMENTS

Make sure you take a multivitamin (see *Resources*). For acute cases, 1 or 2 capsules twice a day; in chronic cases, take 2 capsules after lunch (the time of day when the pancreas tends to be at its weakest). Take **chromium GTF**, chromium picolinate, or liquid chromium. In acute cases, take 100–200mcg 3–4 times per day; for chronic conditions take 200–400mcg once or twice a day. Multiminerals can be taken once or twice a day in acute cases, 1 capsule each time. For chronic conditions, take 2 capsules once a day.

Homeopathic remedy **R86**, the 'blood sugar' drops can be taken, 10 drops every 3–4 hours. For chronic conditions, take 15 drops upon rising and again half an hour after lunch. For women, R20 'glandular drops' can be taken, 15 drops once a day. For men, 15 drops of R19 once a day, first thing in the morning upon rising.

Try using a positive thought for stimulating the pancreas.

'I am expressing positively all my most cherished thoughts and feelings.'

GROUP 21

Water Balance and the Master Hormone Regulator

PHASE FIVE

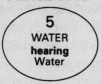

5
WATER
hearing
Water

For guidance on how to use the information in this section see p. 65.

The posterior pituitary regulates the distribution and movement of water in the body, moving the body from acid states to more alkaline states. When the body goes towards the acid side of the cycle, water is retained in the soft tissues and the vital organs. When the body becomes too alkaline, water is withheld. The quantity of water is in direct proportion to the build up of pressure (acidity) and space (alkalinity) inside the body (see p. 14).

At an emotional level, when fluid is stuck, the body moves into a state of grief. Past pains and hurts that have been suppressed and repressed in the body give rise to problems such as bloating, acidity and retention of fluids in the ankles, wrists, stomach and fingers. In the extreme condition, or when there is a genetic metabolic imbalance, the face, hands and feet may enlarge, in a condition known as acromegaly. Acromegaly is the result of a biochemical imbalance between the pituitary and the thyroid. Any overload on the pituitary affects the thyroid gland (see p. 115) and disturbs the acid–alkaline balance, which can lead to excess calcium being excreted. This makes it even more difficult to resolve the energy equation.

When acidity builds up inside the body tissue, fat is produced as a response. If the body becomes too acidic, fats cannot be broken down, since the acidity forms a biochemical barrier to the freeing, utilisation, and absorption of energy from the fat. Cellulite is the trapped fat surrounded by water which is working to neutralise the effects of over-acidity. The body needs to re-ignite the incomplete energy cycles and free the unliberated energy so that the stalled fats, proteins and carbohydrates can be broken down, re-absorbed and utilised. The acidic effect of the environment and of stress prevents the completion of this energy cycle.

Excessive sweating may also result from an imbalance affecting the posterior pituitary, when the body is unable to regulate its thermostat. Hot and cold, sweats are a sign that there is an acid–alkaline imbalance and too much or too little water is building up in the body cavities in general. This condition may be brought about as a result of an excess of toxins and poisonous waste products building up, which the body attempts to get rid of.

The imbalanced pituitary loses its ability to 'track' random objects that may be opposing the body from within and this drastically alters its hormone responses. It is the job of the pituitary to control the body's overall response to internal change via hormones that regulate the water balance on the acid–alkaline scale.

One of the major functions of the pituitary with the hypothalamus is to regulate the hunger response and the satisfaction point. This is a 'set point' within each individual, which is vital because it controls the appetite mechanism. Many people suffering from obesity, anorexia nervosa, bulimia, and other weight or eating disorders have an imbalanced set point. This means that the response of the pituitary and hypothalamus is being over-ridden, so the brain does not get the message to stop (or start) eating. The body's ability to come to a balance, or a resting point of equilibrium, is damaged. Like crying 'wolf' too often, the body is eventually unable to respond or react after the body's chemical 'alarms' have been raised over an extended period.

The set point helps to regulate the basal metabolism, the communication between the hypothalamus and the thyroid. Once disturbed by stress and environmental pollutants, the pituitary will not be chemically coordinated with the thyroid, causing metabolic problems that prevent fats, proteins and carbohydrates from being properly digested and absorbed. Leftover metabolites may then be stored as fat, as is the case with thyroid-based obesity.

FOODS

When Group 21 appears as the first or second number in your questionnaire analysis your water balance is affected and your body is becoming over acidic. Avoid breads with yeast, oranges, grapefruit, cheese, milk, tomatoes, potatoes, peppers, aubergines, spinach, white flour, white sugar, coffee, tea, peanuts, rhubarb, melons. When there is excessive sweating increase your consumption of foods from the Water Phase (Phase Five, see p. 183 and the Five Phase food chart on p. 170). The Water Phase opposes the Fire Phase (Phase Two), so increase water grain and buckwheat, as this may help to reduce sweating. Avoid all the Wood (Phase One) grains and beans and flesh foods as this may promote greater acidity. Eat more vegetables, as their minerals tend to help balance problems affecting the water balance.

SUPPLEMENTS

First and foremost use the tissue salt **Natrum Muricum** (Nat. Mur. 6) to balance water in the body. This comes in 6X potency; 3 tablets can be taken under the tongue every 3 hours for acute problems. For chronic conditions, take 2 tablets upon rising and again before bed. Pituitary problems respond to Evening Primrose. Take 500–1,000mg 1–3 times a day. The herb Agnus Castus is very effective for menopausal/hormonal imbalances; use 500–1,000mg 1–3 times a day. Take a balanced

multivitamin (see *Resources*), once or twice a day, supplemented with vitamin C, 1,000–2,000mg once or twice a day.

Try using a positive thought for stimulating the posterior pituitary.

'I am continually reaching my physical, emotional and spiritual completeness.'

GROUP 22

The Calcium Controller or Parathyroid

PHASE FOUR

4
METAL
smell
Amino acids

For guidance on how to use the information in this section see p. 65.

As part of the thyroid mechanism, the parathyroid regulates the secretion of calcium in the form of calcitonin. The parathyroid also regulates blood clotting by releasing a substance that thickens the blood and stops a wound from bleeding. When the body goes to the extreme acid side of the cycle more calcium is released. Calcium levels that are too high or too low affect the acid–alkaline balance. When calcium levels are disturbed, the density of bone can be affected, soft tissue in the vital organs may harden, and in general things can become too 'brittle' or too 'hard'.

The parathyroid also regulates the iodine and phosphorus levels that balance the 'fire' power of the digestive system. When this mechanism is disturbed the whole conversion of foods into energy is hampered, which therefore affects the absorption of foods and the elimination of waste matter. Any problems with the bones, teeth or vital organs may involve imbalances of the parathyroid. Imbalances affecting the parathyroid also distort how you feel in your body. The body tends to become 'fossilised', graven, solid, heavy, rock-like. The spine and all the limbs may be 'petrified', giving a feeling of carrying the whole weight of the world on the shoulders and back, as with certain types of arthritis and bone troubles.

FOODS
The most important foods to eat when there is a parathyroid imbalance are enzyme-rich foods. In particular, increase all the leafy, dark green vegetables; these are high in enzymes as well as high in calcium. (See Group 10, page 117.)

SUPPLEMENTS
Make sure that you take a well-balanced **multivitamin** (see *Resources*), and the tissue salts calcium phosphate and calcium sulphate. Take 1 tablet of each tissue salt 3 times a day.

From the homeopathic remedies, use **R34**, for building bone tissue. This remedy can be taken 3 times a day – 10 drops for acute cases in half a glass of water. For chronic bone problems take 20–30 drops once a day in water.

Try using a positive thought for stimulating your parathyroid.

'I am liberating myself physically, emotionally and spiritually.'

GROUP 23

The Auto-immune System and the Spleen

PHASE THREE

3
EARTH
taste
Sugars and
carbohydrates

For guidance on how to use the information in this section see p. 65.

When Group 23 appears in your questionnaire analysis it means that there are allergic reactions weakening your auto-immune system. The auto-immune response regulates the way the body responds to an invasion by substances by producing sequences of amino acids that reject any substance that can overwhelm and weaken the body and mind. A healthy auto-immune response can successfully reject and refuse any substance in the air, soil or water, for example, by producing the protein sequence, or antigen pattern. The body appreciates positive or negative qualities in any substance and creates a chemical barrier or boundary to protect the body from any harmful effect.

The spleen is located on the left side of the body under the lower ribs outside the stomach area. It is about half the size of your hand, and is composed of soft tissue. The spleen is vital in the production and managing of white and red cells; it also supports the lymphatics (see p. 160), a primary clearing system for elimination of waste materials. The spleen participates in the elimination of used white and red cells and passes them on to the liver for elimination. It also deals with purified blood, helping the body absorb, assimilate, and utilise food nutrients.

The spleen works with the pancreas and liver to manage and

ensure good healthy blood, getting rid of anything that can antagonise the body in biochemical terms. The foods we eat can either continue the path of destruction, toxicity and poisons, or help relieve and restore the body, keeping it vital, healthy and young.

The emotional manifestations of spleen disorders are seen in the release of negative, acrimonious, disappointed and selfish feelings. This correlates with the physical role of the spleen as a major site for the elimination of waste materials. People who 'vent their spleen' too often are broken, sullen people, trapped in recurring negative thoughts and feelings about themselves and others. Perhaps this is because they cannot say 'no' to the substances that are in fact poisoning them.

Because of the environment and all natural processes being contaminated, the spleen cannot get rid of waste fast enough, or neutralise quickly enough the life-diminishing substances that the body is taking in. This is why children, adolescents and adults today are developing allergies.

Allergies are one of the most misunderstood areas of medicine. This is because most doctors treat allergies by giving them so much power that many sufferers feel disempowered and weakened. As a consequence, the treatment and approach strengthens the allergic reaction. The allergic reaction antagonises the immune and auto-immune systems to such an extent that the body becomes defenceless.

An allergic reaction triggers both a physical/biochemical and a mental/emotional imbalance. They are not separate. An allergic reaction **must** be understood as the epitome of a physical and emotional trauma, shock or injury that triggers something unresolved in a very fundamental way within the individual's constitution. The problem may be genetic, and may have existed for several generations. The body yearns to be better or free and yet at the same time is unable to push away the very substance, that once integrated could restore the body, mind and spirit to a greater sense of well-being and strength. The glands and organs cannot use the temporary invasion to their advantage. They can only react antagonistically to the substance. In short, the body and mind cannot immunise itself.

Allergies can produce numerous physical and psychological symptoms such as sleep disturbances, rashes, asthma, eczema, depression, concentration problems and general poor health. All cases of asthma are in essence allergic reactions rooted in the inability of the individual to find balance, rest and equilibrium. In Oriental medicine the spleen is the root cause of this condition and is related to the inherited family energy, the foundation from which we grow. The biochemical symptoms and unconscious emotionally imbalanced patterns are both part of the picture. There may be a deep sense of rejection which affects the body, weakens the constitution and causes spiritual and emotional suffering.

FOODS
Increase your consumption of millet, sweet potatoes, yams and all squash types. All vegetables and all roots and tubers support the spleen.

SUPPLEMENTS
For acute conditions of allergic reactions, take vitamin A, 15,000–30,000i.u. once or twice a day; **pantothenic acid**, 500–1,500mg once or twice a day; **vitamin C**, 1,000–3,000mg once or twice a day; vitamin E, 400–600i.u. once or twice a day before food, and a **multivitamin** (see *Resources*), 1 or 2 tablets before lunch.

From the homeopathic remedies, use **R93**, 10 drops in half a glass of water 3 times a day.

For chronic conditions use the following: Gamma Linoleic Acid (GLA) 500–1,500mg 1–3 times a day, 1 **multivitamin** tablet (see *Resources*) twice a day, 1 multimineral tablet (see *Resources*) once or twice a day.

From the homeopathic remedies, use **R93**, the immune fortifier, 15 drops twice a day; **R84**, the hayfever drops, 15 drops before bed and **R85**, fungus drops, 15 drops before bed.

Try using a positive thought for stimulating your spleen.

'I am appreciating and enjoying my life fully.'

GROUP 24

The Lymphatic System
PHASE THREE

3
EARTH
taste
Sugars and
carbohydrates

For guidance on how to use the information in this section see p. 65.

When Group 24 appears in your questionnaire analysis it indicates that the lymph glands and lymphatic system are congested, blocked and not functioning properly because of poisons and toxins obstructing the flow of lymph.

The lymphatic system supports the elimination of cellular waste. Dead white cells and other by-products of cell activity drain into the network of lymph channels, which run alongside the veins and arteries. Whereas the blood system works with the pumping action of the heart, the lymph system needs to be stimulated. It works with only the force of gravity, which allows the lymphatic fluids to drain down towards the feet. The major drainage duct for the lymph is located above the nipples, towards the centre of the thorax, and this can be stimulated with massage.

Given the level of toxins and poisons in the environment, the lymphatic system builds up poisonous wastes, causing swelling and enlargement of specific nodes. The major lymph nodes are located in the neck, on both sides of the armpits, and in the groin. The more the nodes swell, the more it indicates that acidity is building up in the body, which in turn starts the flow of mucus as an automatic response. Mucus production is an attempt by the body to protect the mucous membrane. Tenderness, heat, swelling and fever are signs of lymph congestion.

The swelling of a lymph node is a sign that the body will be susceptible to inflammation. This in turn sets the stage for infection. The lymphs carry vital nutrients to the cells as well as helping eliminate bacteria to prevent inflammation, congestion and infection.

Addiction to any stimulant or sedative causes major congestion in the lymph system. Addiction may be to a substance, person, place or thing. Anything can be used addictively when for some reason the individual feels overwhelmed and unable to cope with physical or emotional stress. An individual who feels pain, sorrow or suffering and a feeling of being unfulfilled in day-to-day life, may repeatedly take a substance that gets rid of the pain. However, such repeated use usually leads to feeling trapped and does not give the individual a sense of well-being. All drugs used in excess destroy the individual autonomy of a person because they create dependency. Whatever the physical or emotional pain might be, the drug does not resolve the problem. It may produce temporary relief but the individual loses touch with the original pain, and therefore is less able to resolve the problem. This leads to feeling more and more spiritually barren. Drugs teach the body and mind that the 'being' does not function, this creates an increasing neediness which is rooted in deprivation. On the other hand, addiction may be a desire to rise above the mundane and experience something beyond the ordinary. The problem lies in the fact that the more of the substance one takes, the more the mental and emotional torture.

All concentrated sugars, protein and fats will affect the lymph and may contribute to congestion in the lymph system. Nowhere in body chemistry is this unbalanced equation more evident than how poisonous waste affects the lymph. White flour, white sugar, an abundance of processed foods, and any tendency to over- or under-consume fats, proteins or carbohydrates will immediately affect the flow of lymph. The use of alcohol, tobacco and other drugs such as cocaine, marijuana,

LSD or Ecstasy suggests an inability to cope physically and emotionally.

FOODS

To rejuvenate the lymphatic system, choose the foods that are high in natural enzymes. Enzyme foods are raw leafy vegetables, greens (particularly lettuces), watercress, parsley, mustard and cress, celery. Other particularly good sources are radiccio, escarole, chicory and the herb, rocket. Fresh vegetable juices cleanse and feed the lymph. Use a combination chosen from carrot, celery, parsley, beetroot and watercress. Increase all root vegetables.

Decrease your consumption of oats, rye, bread, fried foods and red meat. Focus your choices on fish and chicken. Avoid pork, ham, sausage, bacon, salamis, oranges, grapefruit, tomatoes, peppers, spinach, cheese, cream, butter, pulses, cakes, candies, biscuits, tea, coffee or sugary drinks.

SUPPLEMENTS

The following vitamins and minerals should be taken as supplements. **Vitamin C**, as calcium or magnesium ascorbate, for acute cases, take 500–1,500mg, 2–3 times a day; in chronic conditions, take 1,000–2,000mg 1–2 times a day. Vitamin B complex, in acute cases, 25–50mg twice a day; in chronic conditions 50–75mg 1–2 times a day; vitamin B12, in acute cases, 1,000–2,000mg 1–3 times a day; in chronic conditions 1,500–3,000mg 1–2 times a day; pantothenic acid, in acute cases, 1,500mg, 1–2 times a day at breakfast and/or lunch; in chronic conditions 2,000mg, 1–2 times a day; also take a multimineral (see *Resources*), in acute cases, 1 capsule 1–3 times a day, in chronic conditions, 1 capsule 2–3 times a day.

From the homeopathic remedies for acute cases of inflammation, take 10 drops of Reckeweg R1 3 times a day, for chronic cases take 20–30 drops once a day before bed. R60 in the same dosages as above will purify the blood. The same dosages again of R26 will drain the lymph and stimulate the defences.

Try using a positive thought for stimulating your lymphatic system.

'I am fulfilled as a total human being.'

Part Four

In our Western tradition we are taught to think in specifically linear terms, putting things in their box and treating them logically. This mindset lends itself to the notion of 'proving things' which we associate with scientific progress. However, it leaves no space for unmeasurable human factors such as feelings.

In Oriental philosophies the whole universe is represented in a big circle that flows, moves and interrelates, including every aspect of life. Please try to open your mind's eye to this other way of understanding the body, mind and spirit.

In introducing the concept of the Five Phases, I have tried to show them as 5 elements interrelating and changing each other, just as every living thing is constantly in a state of flux.

THE FELT FORMULA is about restoring balance within the body. The questionnaire establishes which of the 24 glands and organs of the body have gone out of balance. Each gland and organ is connected to 1 or more of the Five Phases. Once you know where your problem lies and which Phase it relates to, you can follow the Five Phase food chart with the specific instructions for your gland and organ to restore your body to fitness. As a general rule you should always try to eat foods from across the Five Phases.

The Five Phases

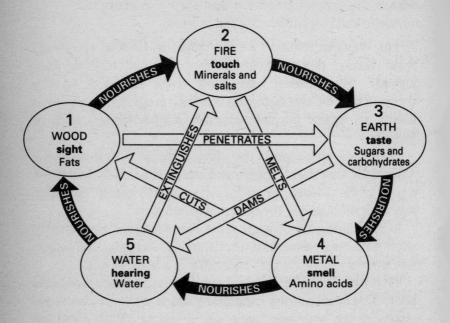

Ancient Chinese tradition describes the Five Phases of nature related to the five elements of Wood, Fire, Earth, Metal and Water. In Indian tradition metal would be referred to as air or ether. Every naturally occurring substance, including the organs and substances of the body, and every food, can be identified with one of these elements.

The chart shows the relationships between the five elements and the organs. The endocrine hormones are related to all the elements, since complex hormone functions are active at each Phase. Each element is also associated with one of the five senses, and with one of the 'building blocks' of nutrition.

METABOLISM

Metabolism involves two complementary sets of reactions – anabolism and catabolism. The catabolic reactions break down substances in the body to release energy, whereas the anabolic reactions build up substances and store energy. The arrows across the centre of the chart depict catabolic reactions, which release energy and create waste in the cycle. The nourishment arrows around the outside of the chart represent the anabolic reactions in the cycle.

NOURISHMENT CYCLE PHASE BY PHASE

ANABOLISM

1 Wood is necessary fuel to make a fire burn.
2 Ash from the fire fertilises, nourishes and supports growth from the earth.
3 Inside the earth metal ore is compressed.
4 Metals feed water in the sea, rivers and oceans in the form of minerals.
5 Water containing minerals (metals) plus earth allows trees (wood) to grow.

CATABOLISM

1 Wood penetrates the earth; trees grow roots into the earth.
2 Fire melts through its heat.
3 Earth dams water.
4 Metal cuts wood.
5 Water extinguishes fire.

ANATOMY BY PHASES

1 Liver and gall bladder
  Sex organs

2 Heart
  Post-pituitary
  Sinus (ears, nose, throat)
  Brain

3 Stomach
  Veins and arteries
  Pancreas
  Spleen
  Lymphatic glands

4 Colon
  Intestines
  Lungs
  Thymus
  Thyroid gland
  Skin
  Parathyroid gland

5 Bones
  Muscles
  Adrenalin
  Kidney

The Five Phase Food Chart

	Phase One	*Phase Two*
Grains & Starches	Barley = Oats – Rye = Wheat –	Corn = Corn on the cob = Popcorn =
Pulses	Fava beans – Green lentils – Mung beans – Split peas –	Red lentils =
Vegetables	Artichoke = Broccoli = Cos lettuce + Courgette = Green beans = Lettuce, green & red + Parsley + Peas, green = Runner beans =	Brussel sprouts – Asparagus = Chicory + Endive = Escarole + Green onions = Okra + Tomatoes – Peppers, red & green –
Fruits	Avocado = Grapefruit – Lemon + Lime + Oranges – Plum = Pomegranate =	Apricots = Guava = Persimmons = Raspberries = Strawberries =

Key
– eat less
= eat in moderation
+ eat more

Phase Three	Phase Four	Phase Five
Acorn squash =	Potato =	Buckwheat +
Butternut squash =	Rice =	
Hubbard squash =		
Millet +		
Sweet potato =		
Yams =		
Chickpeas =	Quorn =	Aduki beans +
	Soya beans =	Black beans =
		Kidney beans +
Aubergine −	Cabbage −	Beetroot =
Parsnip +	Cauliflower −	Curly kale +
Rocket +	Celery =	Hijiki +
Savoy cabbage =	Celeriac =	Mushrooms −
Spinach −	Chinese cabbage =	
Spring Greens =	Garlic =	*Sea Vegetables*
Yellow squash +	Iceberg lettuce −	Kombu +
	Kohlrabi =	Nori +
	Leeks =	Wakame +
	Mustard and cress +	
	Onion =	
	Radish =	
	Swede =	
	Turnip =	
	Watercress +	
	Sea Vegetables	
	Carageen =	
	Dulse +	
Apple =	Peach =	
Banana =	Pear +	
Coconut −	Prunes =	
Dates =	Cherries =	
Figs =		
Grapes −		
Mango +		
Melon =		
Papaya +		
Pineapple =		
Raisins +		

	Phase One	*Phase Two*
Seeds and Nuts	Brazil – Cashew – Peanuts –	Pistachio – Sunflower + Sesame =
Meats	Chicken = Chicken liver –	Wood pigeon = Lamb =
Miscellaneous	Bran = Brandy – Lard – Marmite = Nut butters = Olives and olive oil = Peanuts – Pickles = Vinegar = Yeast –	Beer = Coffee – Chocolate – Tomato sauce – Spirits: vodka = gin – Red wine =
Dairy	Butter – Cream – Mayonnaise – Salad cream – Yoghurt (sweet) +	Mozzarella = Ricotta +
Fish	Clams – Trout =	Lava bread + Langoustine = Prawn = Shrimp =

Key
– eat less
= eat in moderation
+ eat more

Phase Three	Phase Four	Phase Five
Almonds +	Walnuts =	Chestnuts =
Hazel nuts =		
Pecan =		
Pine nuts =		
Pumpkin seeds +		
Pheasant =	Beef –	Ham –
Quail =	Turkey +	Pork –
Rabbit =		Sausage –
		Luncheon meats –
		Salami –
Whisky =	Rum –	Soy sauce =
White wine =		Tamari sauce =
		Sea salt =
Cottage cheese =	Feta cheese =	
Ice cream –	Eggs =	
Milk –		
Yoghurt (sour) +		
Brill +	Cod =	Caviar =
Dover sole +	Herring +	Fish eggs =
John Dory +	Mackerel +	Lobster =
Lemon sole +	Perch =	Mussels =
Salmon =	Plaice =	Octopus =
Swordfish =	Halibut +	Oysters =
Tuna =	Lemon sole +	Roe +
		Sardines =
		Scallops =
		Squid =

The Healing Qualities of Food

Remember the goal is balance; too slow or too quick is not the desired pace when addressing problems of the body through food therapy.

The simplest way to understand the effect of foods on the body is the Five Phase system found in Oriental medicine. Rather than going deeply into the theories and principles of the Oriental theories, it is enough to say that foods can be divided into the 5 groups or Phases by their sedating (Yin) and stimulating (Yang) properties.

The Five Phase chart on p. 170 shows the metabolic relationships between the groups of foods and the glands and organs of the body. To help explain their interaction the Chinese equated each Phase to an element (wood, fire, earth, metal and water) and also to 1 of the 5 senses (sight, touch, taste, smell and hearing). These are explained below.

Once you have worked out your score in the questionnaire, you will know which part of your body is weakened or over-strained. The Glands and Organs notes on p. 69–163 will tell you to increase the foods in some Phases and avoid the foods in others. The chart overleaf lists all the foods by Phase so that you can select your diet without difficulty.

Generally, unless your questionnaire analysis and your treatments from Part Three direct you otherwise, you should aim always to eat a variety of foods. Do not get stuck in eating the same things all the time, since this will tend to lead to deficiencies/excesses as well as cravings/addictions. Balance your choice of grains, beans, raw and cooked vegetables and meats from all the different Phases. Try to avoid eating toxic foods – white flour, white sugar, cakes, biscuits, pastries, soft drinks and junk foods – but allow yourself to eat a little of what you crave. If you then still crave that particular food/taste, locate it on the Five Phase food chart and eat the vegetables from that Phase and the preceding one. For example, if you crave chocolate, from Phase Two eat asparagus, okra and green onions and from Phase One eat green beans and lettuce. By doing this you will be nourishing the Phase and restoring the balance.

Re-programming yourself to healthy eating after years of over-indulgence is not an easy matter! Don't be hard on yourself – if you 'blow it' start again the next day. Above all, don't hold yourself in the guilt of yesterday's mistakes. Take your time, have fun and 'balance your poisons'.

PHASE ONE

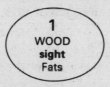

1
WOOD
sight
Fats

Phase One contains the foods of the liver. The liver is the 'planning' organ. It monitors the incoming information, judges how the metabolism is doing and regulates the whole process of nourishment throughout the body. In Chinese medicine the liver, the mid-brain and the eyes are the first parts of the body to be formed after conception. They are therefore believed to be the direct expression of the individual soul or spirit of each person.

Green coloured vegetables strengthen the liver and its powers of detoxification, rejuvenation and transformation. This is because they are high in enzymes which clean up the system.

The liver is connected to the tension or looseness of the muscle fibres. As blood flows into the veins and arteries, this strengthens the heart and the nerves. The heat rising from the lower abdomen regulates the digestion of food. When an individual craves pickles, vinegar, fats and chicken there is an imbalance of the fat metabolism.

High cholesterol, gall-stones, mastitis, lumpy congested lymph nodes, nausea, car-sickness, vomiting, sour abdominal belching, diarrhoea and headaches shortly after eating are all due to a toxic liver not being able to digest. Migraine headaches are often traced back to liver and gall bladder troubles. Headaches can be caused by allergic reactions to wheat, oats, yeast and dried beans and pulses. Where the liver is Yang or contracted, carbohydrates can be left to ferment in the body and fats can go rancid because they haven't been cleaned away.

The answer lies in the green vegetables in Phase One as explained in Group Six on p. 98.

PHASE TWO

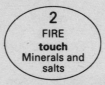

2
FIRE
touch
Minerals and
salts

Phase Two is synonymous with the movement and directing of the blood circulation. The heart moves the blood which contains all the vital nutrients to bath the tissue with fresh nutrients. At the same time, the cells release into the blood carbon dioxide and other by-products of cell energy. These 2 functions are synchronised to give life to the cells of the body and to get rid of the dead waste products. Just like fire, it requires the raw material wood and releases heat in the form of energy. The potential energy of fats, proteins and carbohydrates is ignited via the elements of hydrogen, carbon and nitrogen.

Many of the foods in the second Phase absorb tremendous amounts of sunlight, and often have colours and qualities that resemble fire and sun. **Corn** will strengthen and stimulate the heart. **Sunflower seeds** ground into a powder and added to corn porridge is an excellent food for the heart. **Apricots** and apricot kernels are known to be detoxifying. The kernels contain naturally occurring B17, amydalin, which has been banned as a very controversial substance because of its chemotherapeutic properties. It destroys acid toxic waste in the same way that fire destroys wood.

In Oriental medicine it is known that when there is weakness or a lack of 'Fire' then moisture and mucus accumulate. In turn moisture can be used to extinguish too much 'Fire'. **Okra** or lady's fingers is one of the most healing foods when there is congestion and acidity. It must be cooked well. Its gelatinous qualities coat, absorb and neutralise acid waste through the digestive tract.

Asparagus, **chicory**, **endive** and **escarole** all have the bitter taste that indicate the supreme 'Fire' foods. After eating asparagus the strong smell of urea in the urine is a sign of the cleansing powers of the asparagus.

In a damp cold climate, if taken in excess the members of the 'night-shade' family, **tomatoes**, **potatoes** and fresh **peppers**, will weaken the heart and the circulation as well as the elimination system. In Mediterranean countries where there is dry heat these foods help the body cope with excessive temperatures and also prevent the rapid loss of vital salt fluids. Excessive consumption of tomatoes and peppers will produce calcium build-up in the veins, arteries, joints and muscles. In countries such as Britain these 'night-shade' foods coupled with too much alcohol, tobacco, spirits and meats are culprits for rheumatism, gout and arthritis. Moderate consumption will never cause problems but in excess they will always cause circulation problems leading to cold hands and feet.

Phase Two foods taken in excess are over-stimulating. When there are cravings for alcohol, coffee, chocolate, tobacco, the abuse substances of modern societies, there is an imbalance of the heart which creates a profound sense of lack, lack of love, lack of self-acceptance and guilt. The more one takes of these foods the more there will be a sense of something missing and the worse the addiction becomes.

Group Two of the Glands and Organs section on p. 76 deals directly with problems with the heart.

PHASE THREE

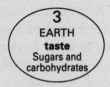

Virtually everybody is deficient to a certain degree in Phase Three because the Earth Phase concerns how much energy you have, both emotionally and physically. The focus of this Phase is on the digestion – the stomach, the pancreas and the spleen. The flavour of sweetness seems to be most people's major craving. The immediate oral gratification of something sweet gives people the feeling that they have more energy and there the sugar addiction begins.

By eating more of the sweet vegetables in Phase Three and avoiding fruit or refined sugars, you can bring your pancreas which regulates the blood sugar back into balance. Also make sure you eat green leafy vegetables at least once a day as well as cooked green vegetables.

There is an important psychological imbalance related to sugar addiction. The physical energy loss may indicate unhappiness and a sense of defeatism or a suppression of negative emotions. Try to discover where these negative feelings are springing from then focus on the positive aspects of your own self-worth. (See p. 91 and 149 for positive thoughts needed by Group 4 and Group 20.) Eat more sour tasting things as they may help to balance the craving for sweets. Appreciate the other foods that will really provide and produce the stability that you want from your foods and life in general.

Millet is known to most people as budgie seed but it is one of the oldest known cultivated grains. Many of the Egyptian pharaohs were buried with millet in their sarcophagi. It was believed that millet was created for the Gods. It has many wonderful properties. Most importantly, it is the only alkalising grain. It neutralises acidity and toxins in the digestion and helps clear the lymphatic system.

Millet has 7 of the 8 essential amino acids in an excellent balance. The Swiss use it to promote beautiful lustrous hair but I believe that everybody should start eating millet to improve their physical appearance, energy levels and emotional balance. It is very easy to digest and helps the digestion of other foods. Millet cream is known to cure duodenal ulcers, colitis and irritable bowel syndrome amongst many other problems. Unfortunately millet is not yet generally available in supermarkets. You will have to find it in health food shops but it is not expensive. Millet is cooked just like rice. Simmer for 30 minutes with two cups of water for every cup of millet.

Jerusalem artichokes are another very valuable Phase Three food. They help to stimulate the production of insulin and are very good for people who are allergic to wheat. **Green chard** or **Ruby chard** is one of my favourite green vegetables. The leaves have a long whitish stem running vertically through them. Chopped and steamed like spinach, chard tastes wonderful and is excellent for you. Steamed and blended in a mixer, it makes a super recover soup that will get into your system quickly, restoring the blood sugar and energy levels.

Like chard, **yellow squash** is very high in all the important life-giving minerals and vitamins: vitamin A, calcium, potassium, magnesium and phosphorus. Jerusalem artichokes, chard and squash are a good replacement for those who eat too much bread. Although not well known in Britain, all the different types of squash are very good sources of carbohydrate energy.

Rather like potatoes, they are very satisfying baked because of their taste.

Aubergine is another member of the 'night-shade' family mentioned in Phase Two. This should not be eaten during cold and wet weather or if there are any acid problems in the digestion, bones or muscles (arthritis and rheumatism).

Parsnips are one of the tastiest Phase Three foods. Baked in the oven they caramelise enough to satisfy the real sugarholic. The same goes for **sweet potatoes** or yams. Parsnips are packed with carbohydrate energy, vitamin A, calcium and are very high in potassium.

The fruits of Phase Three are very good and all very sweet. When Phase Three is out of balance, fruit can be eaten every other day for breakfast and lunch or as a snack between lunch and dinner. No more than 3 pieces of fruit should be eaten per day as this will cause blood sugar problems. Dried fruit should be avoided as the sugar content is too high.

One of the popular misconceptions among raw food faddists is that you can eat as much fruit as you want. This is definitely not the case. If there is any bloating in the stomach, headache, energy problem or skin trouble avoid fruit and eat only 2 pieces every few days.

In general fruit is for warm, dry, sunny weather. It replaces mineral-salts due to loss of fluids in heat. When the weather is damp or cold, raw fruit will make the body very cold. Fruit can be used for detoxification purposes, otherwise the key word is moderation. If you eat fruit that would grow seasonally, you will usually be on the right track.

Bananas are the exception to the rule. Avoid them if your digestion is upset but otherwise they are good all year round. The other exception is **papaya** or paw-paw which has remarkable powers to heal stomach upsets, especially acidity. Papaya sooth any inflamed mucous membrane in the stomach or bowels.

In Phase Three **oranges** and **grapefruits** should be avoided. It is a myth that these fruits are good for slimming!

Small amounts of **almonds, pumpkin seeds, hazelnuts** and **pine nuts** are very good (if you tend not to chew well you should grind them in a coffee grinder). Avoid eating more than 3oz (90g). Nuts are very concentrated and high in fats. It is easy to eat too many which will lead to wind and a swollen stomach.

Dairy products are the subject of much controversy. Lots of diet books tell people they are allergic to dairy products but to me a healthy person can eat the right amount of *all* foods. Dairy products are no exception unless of course you have had a tested and confirmed reaction.

The benefits of **yoghurt** outweigh any ideas of allergy. If it contains live bacteria (acidophilus, caucausius, bifidus, thermadolphilus etc) it can restore balance in many types of digestive and bowel upsets. If you have been avoiding this food, believing it isn't suited to you, the way to re-train your stomach to be able to digest it is to take half a teaspoonful in a glass of water. A glass of water with 1/2–2 teaspoonsful of yoghurt and a tiny pinch of sea salt will cure severe indigestion in 10 minutes much better than any over-the-counter digestive tablet!

Ice cream is so high in cane sugar it should only be eaten occasionally as a treat.

Cottage cheese is very easy to digest and is an excellent source of protein. In general it is best to avoid **milk** apart from small amounts in tea or coffee or in cooking. The myth of calcium in milk must be put to rest. The calcium in pasteurised milk has been enriched and therefore will not be utilised by the body. Unpasteurised milk from sanitary sources may be an exception.

Salmon and **tuna**, whether fresh or canned, are both wonderful proteins for Phase Three. Grilled or baked fish with a little olive oil, lemon juice and herbs cooked to perfection is delicious!

Pheasant or **quail** are traditional British foods that are delicious and nutritious. Rich creamy or fruity sauces should only be eaten occasionally, sorry! But you can sauté the game first in the pan with a drop of oil and garlic, onions, salt and pepper and then grill or bake with rosemary or thyme which is a great compensation.

PHASE FOUR

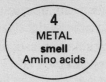

Phase Four is linked with respiration. The Chinese use of the word 'metal' refers to the chemical elements such as hydrogen, carbon and oxygen which are present in air. In the Indian tradition Phase Four would be referred to as the air or ether Phase but the Chinese see the chemical elements in the air as solid or fixed, hence the word 'metal'.

When the metal elements are disturbed, breathing will therefore be affected. One of the first signs of fear is fast shallow breathing, and an imbalance in Phase Four exaggerates emotions which often leads to fearfulness. Phase Four also controls the large intestine.

Metaphorically speaking, when fire consumes the fuel wood and burns the earth, metals are freed. Excessive Phase Three troubles (very high blood sugars) will eventually begin to disturb metal Phase Four or bring it out of balance.

Virtually everybody with respiratory illness such as coughs, asthma, bronchitis or emphysema have too much acid in their systems. Skin problems are also a sign of this. People with these problems often have very tight muscles, they are impulsive fast thinkers and have either too much moisture or too little in their lungs and sinuses. Either way this indicates a Phase Four imbalance.

When breathing is stifled rather than fresh and clear the lungs are out of balance and the exchange of oxygen and carbon dioxide is not in rhythm. Waste will build up in the intestines reducing the assimilation of food. Intestinal disturbances are very common and often they are caused by environmental poisoning when heavy metals are deposited on the membranes of the lungs and large intestine.

Rice is the premier grain of Phase Four. In Oriental medicine rice was thought to be a gift from the 'gods of Heaven'. Macrobiotic diets suggest eating rice every day but in Britain where the weather is damp and cold, this is too much rice. Excess cattarrh and constipation are signs that you are eating too much rice which may bring on cravings for sweets, tobacco and alcohol.

When Phase Four is disrupted **beef** should most definitely be reduced. **Turkey** is a good alternative as is **tofu** or **tempeh** (this is a Balinese fermented soybean dish available from health food shops). Reduce the consumption of **potato, cabbage, cauliflower** and **cucumber.** Increase **Chinese cabbage, celery, watercress, mustard** and **cress, leeks, radishes, turnips** and **turnip greens. Onions, garlic** and **ginger** should be taken in moderation as should locally grown **lettuces.**

PHASE FIVE

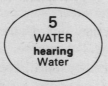

5
WATER
hearing
Water

The Fifth Phase is the Water Phase which is concerned with filtering the blood and elimination of waste via the kidneys and bladder. The temperature of the body varies according to the water content and this in turn is affected by the acidity or alkalinity of the body fluids.

When the body is too acid and waste is building up in the tissues, water cannot be excreted and swelling or bloating occurs. Often the person will feel very cold and will particularly suffer at night with cold hands and feet. They may feel sluggish because too much water disrupts the even distribution or flow of energy. Often there is a feeling of fear and panic attacks are common with Phase Five problems.

Calcium and magnesium are vital to restore balance when the body swings to extremes due to over-acidity (fluid retention) or over-alkalinity (dryness or lack of fluids). Phase Two foods can help because they are high in potassium.

Buckwheat is the grain of the Water Phase. Very popular amongst people from Eastern Europe as well as Japan, kasha or buckwheat groats are a delicious and nutritious food. It is called the winter grain because it provides fast energy and heats up the whole body including the blood.

Soba is a pasta noodle made from pure buckwheat. Sometimes the buckwheat is mixed with wheat which makes **Udon noodles**. Both of these can be cooked like ordinary pasta. They are very delicious although a little more sticky than pasta.

Aduki beans, **kidney beans** and **pinto** are recommended when Phase Five is out of balance. All of these are high in minerals, particularly potassium.

All sea vegetables are in the Phase Five foods. I can't emphasise the potential importance and nutritional value of having them in the diet strongly enough. They contain enormous amounts of protein which is almost pre-digested and so is very easy on the digestion. The minerals in these vegetables are wonderfully healing for anyone suffering from stomach upset, kidney or bladder troubles. They are high in naturally utilisable sodium so can be taken in small amounts by people on salt restricted diets without harm or fluid retention problems.

Many people are horrified by the idea of eating sea vegetables but as a garnish or small portion with a meal or salad they can be marinated and served in many different and delicious ways. I marinate them with lemon juice, basil, oregano, garlic, cumin, salt and pepper and a little olive oil. You can try one at a time, **arami**, **hijiki**, **wakame**, **dulse** or **nori**. Nori comes in sheets and is popular in Japanese food rolled up with rice which is called **Maki**. Toasted and crushed, nori really enhances salad, soup or vegetables. **Kombu** comes in slightly thicker dried pieces and can be added to soups or cooked with any dried beans.

When cooking sea vegetables you should take a very small amount (they swell 7–10 fold during soaking) and soak it in a lot of cold water for half an hour to an hour. You can use boiling water if you are in a hurry. Pour off the water (which makes good plant food) and rinse well in a colander to wash off any residual grit. Then marinate.

Irish moss or **carrageen** has been taken for hundreds of years to treat arthritis and as a tonic and immune strengthener but **kelp** is probably the best known sea vegetable because of its use as an iodine supplement.

The other Phase Five vegetables are **beetroots**. These are a very cleansing food for the kidneys. They contain quite high quantities of vitamin A, potassium and magnesium.

For the summer months, all the **berries** except strawberries and raspberries are Phase Five foods. Berries are very cleansing to the kidneys and bladder as are **watermelon** but they all cool the body so should only be eaten when in season locally.

All the **shellfish** other than clams and shrimps belong to the water element of foods. Shellfish are scavengers and they absorb all the waste and toxic pollutants in our seas and oceans. Very high in iodine and other minerals they should only be taken occasionally. Anyone with degenerative disease or thyroid problems should avoid them entirely.

The flavour of the Water Phase is salty. **Pork, ham, salami** and **luncheon meats** are all Phase Five foods. Much has been written about the harmful effect of salt on the heart and circulatory system. Try not to add salt to your foods. Experiment and stop taking salt for a month, then try it again. Then avoid it for 6 months. By this time you will have overcome your addiction to salt and at the same time restored your taste buds. Use *only* sea salt. **Soy sauce** is an excellent substitute to use in small amounts in cooking. Or **miso** is a concentrated paste which contains natural and healthy bacteria which will help restore the Ph in the intestines. Miso can be used by people who can't take yoghurt to balance intestinal bacteria. Unfortunately in Britain the mass manufacturing of different soy products hasn't yet caught on. They have great value in dietary therapy as long as you take them in moderate and appropriate amounts.

The Use of Supplements: Vitamins and Minerals

Using supplements to your diet can counteract the problems of modern life but they are not a panacea. A concentrated quantity of any food has its effect on the body's balance and supplements should only be taken in the quantities and combinations suggested in this book or as directed by a nutritionist.

The following is a guide to the role of each vitamin and mineral, their natural sources and optimal supplementation levels. Each vitamin or mineral needs to be balanced in the body by an opposite element.

Taken in an informed and careful way, supplements are necessary inconveniences if you want to remain healthy in the modern environment. The risks of degenerative disease increase dramatically if a balanced diet and correct supplementation are not taken.

Medical research has largely ignored the value of minerals and vitamins as supplements in favour of finding drugs to suppress the body's symptoms. Many of the recommended daily intake levels are lower than the ideal. This is especially true in cities where the pollution and stress levels affect the body's ability to absorb nutrients from food.

It is important to take the right brand of supplement as many are made from poor quality materials or contain anti-nutrients such as unnecessary salt, sugar, colours and additives, which prevent the utilisation of the supplement at cell level. The names and addresses of those companies whose products I have tested in my clinical practice and can recommend for the high standards are listed (see *Resources*).

The great debate about natural and synethetic supplements needs clarification. Simply, each nutrient, once isolated, needs to be bonded in a particular way to guarantee that it will travel across the intestinal barriers through which vitamins and minerals have to go in order to be absorbed and utilised. If these individual supplements are not correctly constructed, they are excreted mostly through the urine or bowel waste. Biochemists study the structures of these substances in an attempt to duplicate a strand of them in their natural state as they exist in food or the way they exist naturally in our bodies. A combination of synthetic with natural is an absolute must – and a balance of these increases their effectiveness.

Taking mega-doses of vitamins changes your body chemistry and should only be done under guidance from a trained practitioner.

VITAMINS

Vitamin A is essential for optimal vision, teeth, hair and especially good skin. Recent research has also shown how important vitamin A can be as an anti-cancer factor along with zinc, vitamin C and selenium. Vitamin A's role as anti-infection immune strengthener has now become well established, as has its role as an anti-oxidant. Vitamin A supports the thymus gland as part of the immune system's response. Because of its association with the thymus gland, this vitamin may also be helpful when there is a severe allergic reaction. Vitamin A acts as an anti-histamine.

Vitamin A promotes mucous membranes and other soft tissues. Basic protein absorption and utilisation is supported by vitamin A. Most of vitamin A is stored in the liver.

With less than the optimal amount, individuals may develop inflammations, infections, increased allergic reaction, weakened auto-immunity, night blindness due to low formation of 'visual purple'. Skin, eyes, hair and mucous membrane are all affected areas. This vitamin is best taken in either pre-digested (micolized) liquid form or as beta-carotene. Taken in this form, Vitamin A, which is normally a fat soluble vitamin, becomes soluble in water.

Vitamin A is found in all kinds of liver, especially fish liver, beef, milk and all green vegetables. One very good natural source of vitamin A, retinol, is found in carrots, beets, broccoli, watercress, and mustard and cress.

Optimal dosages recommended: Children 2–10 years 2,000–5,000i.u., 10–15 years old, 5,000–10,000i.u., 15 years and older, 15,000–25,000i.u. These amounts apply to water soluble forms of vitamin A. Doses of more than 100,000i.u. of vitamin A are not recommended unless under the supervision of a doctor. Present UK RDA is 2,500i.u. which is very low for optimal health purposes.

B complex vitamins   A series of water-soluble vitamins that play a vital role in good health for the nervous system, the energy system, the endocrine system and the immune system. These series of vitamins play a vital role essential for growth, energy, stamina-endurance, a strong heart, healthy hair and skin, good digestion and a balanced nervous system.

Mostly derived and grown from yeast-cells and yeasty type extracts, vitamin B complex is found in foods such as whole grains, beans (pulses), liver and all dairy products. The B complex co-enzymes are: B1 thiamin, B2 riboflavin, B3 niacin, B5 pantothenic acid, B6, B12, folic acid, biotin, choline, para-amino benzoic acid (PABA) and inositol. Because they are so inter-dependent, an imbalance in one of these essential vitamins requires attention and supplementation of possibly all of them. A person with less than optimal levels of B complex may develop: anaemia and other red-cell forming troubles, digestive upsets, energy problems – fatigue and lethargy, sleep troubles, weight problems or nervous disorders. Most importantly, the B vitamins support the nerve coating, or myelin sheath and therefore play an essential role in combating stress and its effect on the nerves themselves. In so doing the B vitamins combat and protect us from environmental pollution and toxic wastes.

B1 – thiamin helps the release of energy from carbohydrates. This vitamin is essential for the nerves, healthy digestion, a balance in the hunger and appetite. When there is a deficiency, mental symptoms become pronounced; anxiety, nervousness, irritability, exhaustion and confusion ensue. Various cramps, numbness, tingling, a general inability to cope with stress, and depression also accompany deficiencies. Severe deficiency causes beri-beri. Current RDA levels are: 2.0mg for men, 1.0mg for women.

Recommended levels for optimal health are: 25–100mg daily for men, 20–125mg for women. This is due to the reproductive system requiring higher amounts, especially under stress. Food sources are: all nuts, brewer's yeast, brown rice, wheat, fish, meat and molasses.

B2 – riboflavin is very important in the release of energy from food and plays a vital role in the utilisation of oxygen through the respiratory system. It acts as an 'emergency' vitamin, when stress demands energy from stored fats, B2 helps the release. B2 prevents and counteracts afternoon fatigue and blood sugar lows that produce a 'spaced-out' sensation. General slowness, bowel or digestive upsets, areas of redness on the skin, skin sores and fissures and bone or muscle problems may be symptoms of B2 deficiency. Current RDA levels are: 1.6mg for men, 1.3mg for women. Optimal levels are: 20–100mg for men, 15–85mg for women (higher levels for women 1 week before, and during menstruation). Eggs, cheese, pulses, offal, yoghurt, nuts, seeds and molasses are good food sources of B2.

B3 – niacin is essential for the release of energy from fat and the re-stimulation of 'fat burning'. This vitamin prevents the skin condition, pellagra. Niacin may be a very useful agent for detoxifying the body after extreme trauma or deep emotional injury. Its application for some types of schizophrenia and other mental illness is well documented in the psychiatric journals of nutritional medicine. Niacin has the capacity to stimulate 'incomplete energy' in the body. Niacin can help flush 'heavy metals' and radiation out of soft tissue or fat cells. Niacin is helpful in the treatment of cellulite. It also builds up the ability to cope with stress. Muscular weakness and fatigue, nervous problems and skin troubles are signs of deficiency. Current RDA levels are: 18mg for men, 15mg for women. Any supplement over 25mg may cause bright red flushing and an itchy skin. Doses of 100mg or less are suggested initially until a toleration is reached. Higher doses may promote 'leaching' of other minerals. If you use niacin during a detoxification programme, all other vitamin and mineral levels must be maintained.

B5 – pantothenic acid one of the most under-rated and important vitamins for treating stress, B5 is essential for the healthy functioning of the adrenal glands. B5 promotes the release of energy from fats and carbohydrates. It is an important immune booster and links the immune and energy functions, helping to maintain the body during the 'fight or flight' phase of stress. B5 works as a natural steroid and as an anti-inflammatory nutrient, combating inflammatory arthritis (rheumatoid and osteoarthritis). B5 is essential for avoiding low blood sugar, low energy problems. B5 may be an important key to preventing premature ageing.

Brewer's yeast, wheat germ, nuts, seeds, pulses, whole grain cereals, molasses and eggs are all high in B5. No RDA has been established, but it is estimated to be 3–7mg daily. Optimal health ranges: 100–1,000mg daily. High doses of up to 3g daily have had no documented side effects.

B6 – pyridoxine works as a central activator for protein metabolism and fat metabolism. It is required for healthy growth and a strong nervous system. B6 protects against degenerative heart, nerve and muscle diseases. It helps regulate fluids and mediates potassium and sodium and may have a diuretic-like role that supports the work of the kidneys. Useful in treating acute and chronic nerve and muscle conditions, including Carpal Tunnel Syndrome. This vitamin supports red cell growth and development. It also helps promote weight loss.

Deficiencies cause weakness, anaemia, skin trouble, anxiety and irritability, weight problems and nervous disorders. Vitamin B6 is found in liver, pulses, grains, wheat germ, bananas, avocados, molasses, milk, walnuts, soybeans, carrots and all green leafy vegetables.

There is no UK RDA. In the US, RDA levels are: 1.5–2.2mg daily for men, 0.3–1.7mg for infants and 2.5mg for pregnant/ lactating women. Optimal daily intake: 25–100mg daily as pyridoxyl-5-phosphate only.

B12 — cyanocobalamin is associated with a specific anaemia. It is an essential co-enzyme for protein utilisation. The vitamin is always a first consideration when there is digestive cramping, or an absorption problem. Vital for the formation of red cells and nutrient transportation to the cells, it is vital as well to support the elimination of cellular waste. A 'balancing' vitamin in both front line offence and defence. Supplementation is usually required in vegetarian diets, unless careful dietary information and sources of B12 are well known.

Deficiencies cause severe bowel, gut and intestinal problems and megalobiastic anaemia or pernicious anaemia. Vitamin B12 is found in red meats, fish, eggs, cottage cheese, organ meats, watercress, curly kale, spinach, spirulina, chlorella and sea vegetables such as hijiki, nori, kombu, wakame, arami, carrageen and dulse. The RDA is set at 2mcg. Optimal daily intake: 25–5,000mcg.

Folic acid This is important to support the hormones and the Endocrine system. Vital in protein formation of DNA and RNA, which means that it prevents ageing. Essential for healthy intestines, digestion and a vital link for red cell factors promoting growth. More and more studies show that folic acid may be able to prevent Down's syndrome.

The RDA is set at 300mcg. Research shows that 800mcg is needed during pregnancy. Optimal daily intake: in general, 400mcg–1.4mg.

Choline   plays an essential role in the release of energy from fat and the transportation of energy to the cells, releasing and preventing fat build-up. As a component of lecithin, choline works with other fat-soluble vitamins, transporting and releasing energy. Vital to the brain and neurotransmission, choline is needed for clear thinking, memory and re-call. Choline is also a useful agent in reducing calcium in the plaque that forms in veins and arteries. It reduces the risk of heart disease. A must for heavy drinkers to help aid and support the liver and gall bladder. It prevents cirrhosis.

Food sources are liver, organ meats and grains – especially rice and wheat germ.

No UK RDA exists. The US RDA is 50–200mcg. Optimal daily intake: 100–300mg daily. Larger amounts can be taken for Alzheimer's disease and senility. For clearing fat and debris from veins and arteries use phosphitdyl choline only.

Biotin known as vitamin H   As a co-enzyme and water soluble vitamin, biotin plays a vital role in the 'splitting' phase of fats, proteins, and carbohydrate metabolism. Because of this, biotin has always played an important role in cases of hair loss, alopecia, patch-baldness and scalp-related dermatitis. Biotin is useful in any sports activities to stimulate the muscle-nerve activity. Loss of appetite, fatigue, mental slowness and drowsiness may be helped by supplementing biotin.

Biotin is found in pulses – especially lentils, liver, egg yolk, brewer's yeast and brown rice. Biotin is synthesised in the intestinal flora and can be taken with acidophilus or another live yoghurt.

There is no RDA in the UK. In the US, the RDA is 100–200mcg. Optimal daily intake: 400mcg–1.2mg.

PABA (para-amino benzoic acid)   Often used as a softener and stabilising agent in lotions and hand cream, it can also be taken internally to protect the skin from ultra violet light and harmful radiation from the environment. This role has yet to be fully appreciated. By its close working relationship with folic acid, PABA stimulates the production of intestinal flora which manages the acidity level in the colon. (Some believe this is not a utilisable vitamin separate from its known relationship with folic acid). PABA also stimulates the immune system and works closely with zinc to clear the body of invading bacteria, viruses and antigens. PABA helps the auto-immune response. It is also a co-factor in the formation of red cells.

PABA is found in yeast products, wheat germ, molasses, eggs and yoghurt. It is essential to take PABA as a supplement during courses of chemotherapy or radiotherapy for cancer. PABA is excellent for treating every skin disorder, especially lupus ertythemia, rosacea, hives and allergic skin reactions.

There are no set RDA in the UK or US. Optimal preventative dosages: 80–100mg.

Inositol   Like choline, inositol prevents accumulation of fat in the liver. Together they emulsify and degrade saturated fats, and work with unsaturated fatty acids. Together they also maintain a balance between fats and proteins as they are broken down and utilised. These two agents may prevent hardening of the arteries, kidneys and liver. Large amounts of inositol are found in the analysis of brain tissue. It aids memory, concentration, circulation, nourishes the scalp and hair and helps bowel functions. Inositol has been used successfully in weight management.

There is no RDA in the UK or US. Safe dosages: 200–400mg. Even doses higher than 1,000mg a day have shown no side effects.

Vitamin C More has been written about vitamin C than probably any other vitamin. The truth is that vitamin C will help any and every disease. Principally, vitamin C is necessary for the formation of collagen, connective tissue, skin, cartilage, tendon, muscle, nerves and any protein-based matter in the body. Vitamin C supports all cell-life. By stimulating the immune response, auto-immunity and the energy and endocrine response, it has anti-inflammatory and anti-infection potential. Vitamin C stimulates the movement of cell-waste through the lymphatic drainage system. It is an excellent antidote to many harmful side effects of prescription drugs and antibiotics. Vitamin C should be used at the first signs of colds, congestion or catarrh. It is also an excellent natural 'anti-histamine' for treating the secondary symptoms of hay fever. Vitamin C prevents scurvy. Vitamin C may help detoxify radiation stored in the bowels and soft tissue.

All fresh fruits and fresh vegetables contain vitamin C.

The UK RDA is set at 30mg. In the US the RDA is 60mg. Optimal daily intake: 1,000mg upwards. The symptom of an overdose is irritability of the whole alimentary canal including the bowel. Discontinue the high dosage for 24 hours. Begin again by taking half the dose.

Vitamin D This is one of the fat-soluble vitamins. It is known as the sunshine vitamin because ultra-violet light builds up vitamin D stores at the skin surface. Most important for the formation of healthy bones, teeth, nails, gums and hair. This vitamin works with the absorption of calcium into the intestinal tract. Vitamin D also helps the transport of calcium to the cells and to the bones. The vitamin works best when taken with vitamin A and vitamin E. A deficiency of vitamin D affects the eyes, bones and muscles.

RDA in the UK is 400i.u. for growing children and 100i.u. for adults. Optimal daily intake: 400–800i.u. All dairy products contain this vitamin but it is destroyed in the pasteurisation process.

Vitamin E   A fat-soluble vitamin. Vitamin E is known for its powerful anti-oxidant role. Known as a 'free radical' fighter, vitamin E collects the harmful substances that are absorbed from pollution. Considerable controversy about vitamin E has developed because it has been historically associated with helping stimulate and support fertility and sexual performance. Skin health as well as nerve function is helped by vitamin E. This vitamin is known to reduce inflamed and congested mastoid glands as well as inflamed mastitis. It is an excellent vitamin to take before and after any surgery. New research has shown that vitamin E may have applications in treating cancer and may also be able to be taken as a prevention for cancer. In conjunction with vitamins A, C, B1 and vitamin F, vitamin E slows down the ageing process. Selenium, magnesium and manganese are compatible supplements to take with vitamin E. Vitamin E can soften newly formed scar tissue and prevent hard scarring if used immediately after surgery. Deficiencies may lead to rupturing, haemorrhaging, wasting muscle diseases and high levels of fat cells.

Vitamin E is found in wheat germ, vegetables, liver and other organ meat, sunflower seeds, parsley, broccoli and herring. The UK RDA is not established. In the USA the RDA is 4–6i.u. for infants, 7–13i.u. for children, 15i.u. for adult males and 12i.u. for adult women. Optimal daily intake: 400–1,000i.u. There are several strains of vitamin E, the D-alpha tocopherol, is the most effective for therapeutic use. Take the vitamin in a dry form as succinate.

Vitamin K   Another fat-soluble vitamin, vitamin K is necessary for the formation of prothrobin which helps to coagulate the blood. This vitamin is formed by intestinal bacteria or by petrification. Deficiency causes bleeding and bruising because of the collapse of the capillaries structure and arterial walls.

This vitamin is found in leafy green vegetables, yoghurt,

molasses, safflower oil and some varieties of lettuce and cabbage.

There is no RDA in the UK. Optimal daily intake is: 12–20mcg for infants, 15–100mcg for children and 300–500mcg for adults.

Vitamin P (Bioflavoniods)   Considered as a separate vitamin, P is really part of the C complex. Because of its effectiveness in strengthening the walls of the capillaries, it is used as a preventative treatment for easy bruising. Vitamin P is helpful in severe menstrual problems. It is most used for treating infections, dental troubles and haemmorrhoids. It is particularly helpful in treating weak, receding and bleeding gums.

Found in the fruit pulps of oranges, grapefruit, lemon, plums, cherries and grapes.

There is no RDA in the UK. 200–500mg is effective for treatment for 30 days. There are no known toxic reactions.

Pangamic Acid (B15)   Incorrectly known as vitamin B15, it is a co-factor of the B complex vitamins. It is also known as DMG, calcium pangamate and dimethylglycine. A biochemical intermediary of almost all known functions including hormones, enzymes and neurotransmitters. B15 increases the oxygen to the cells. It is known to reduce the effects of stress and pollution. It also helps strengthen the cardiovascular system and may help lower cholesterol and low-density lipids and triglycerides. There is evidence to support B15 working with chromium to stabilise blood sugar levels.

There is no RDA in the UK. 230–500mg is safe without any known toxic effect.

MINERALS

Calcium   This mineral is necessary for healthy bones and also for balance in the central nervous system. Another form of calcium, calcitonin, is secreted by the parathyroid gland. This prevents calcium levels from going too high. Calcium is the most important mineral to combat acidity. It neutralises the effect of 'too much acid'. Digestive and intestinal acidity causes 'pressure' in the body in general, and this can greatly be reduced by taking calcium prophylactically, creating more a feeling of 'space'. Calcium is an 'alkalising' mineral. Taking calcium aids the transmission of nerve and muscle impulses. Stress and daily life requires supplementing with calcium, especially in women past the age of menstruation. Deficiencies of calcium may lead to digestive, energy, bone, muscle and hormonal troubles. Calcium plays a vital 'go between' role in numerous metabolic processes.

Foods high in calcium are all dairy products (although pasteurisation destroys the utilisable nature of calcium), watercress, carrots, broccoli, oat groats, Horsetail (the herb) and parsley.

The UK RDA is 400–600mg for women and 500–700mg for men. Optimal daily intake: 700–1,200mg for women over 15 years old, 500–1,000mg for men and 200–500mg for children 2–14 years old. Deficiency of calcium causes rickets, sleep troubles, increased pain/inflammation or arthritis and related degenerative bone diseases, muscle weakness or co-ordination problems, mental slowness and stomach and intestinal troubles. During menopause, women urgently need to supplement their diet with calcium as its relationship with oestrogen is disturbed at this time.

Chlorine Essential mineral for regulating the acid-alkaline balance of minerals in blood. Chlorine is an active regulator of the digestive system and of the production of hydrochloric acid. Chlorine helps balance and 'hold' fluids in the right suspension. Too little chlorine will affect the digestion. Too high chlorine will affect the circulation because of fluid imbalance.

Cheese, kippers, watercress, herring, carrots, potatoes and celery all contain ample amounts of chlorine.

There is no RDA in the UK or the US for chlorine.

Chromium plays a vital role in regulating pancreatic and insulin function. It adjusts and regulates the blood sugar levels or the energy 'set-point'. Regular supplementing of chromium helps all the glands and organs increase their energy potential and the ability to withstand stress from the environment. Chromium also helps the breakdown of fats. The 'trivalent' form of chromium is less toxic and therefore more easily absorbed. In the organic form of trivalent chromium bound to nicotinic acid it is transported more readily through the gut. Chromium also helps the breakdown of fats.

Brewer's yeast, fish, wheatgerm, liver, molasses, eggs and cheese supply chromium in the diet. There is no UK RDA for chromium. Optimal and safe doses are: 200–600mcg. 200mcg taken with breakfast and lunch. Do not take more than 600mcg maximum per day as chromium will interfere with the absorption of other vitamins.

Cobalt is an 'activator and carrier' of all the heavy metals: nickel, iron, zinc and selenium. Each of these elements helps in the transport of nutrients that make up red blood cells. This function has only been recognised by studying the medieval and ancient alchemy. Cobalt also has the ability to 'transmute' amino acids. The function of cobalt as a key regulator of acid–alkaline balance has not been recognised or understood. When cobalt is out of balance the entire mind and body link is disturbed. Distorted visions and hallucinations result from a disturbance to the balance of cobalt.

Greens, organ meats and fish are high in cobalt. Healthy soil contains cobalt. Supplementation with doses of cobalt should only be considered in homeopathic form.

The UK RDA is not established.

Copper works in relationship to the immune systems and the thymus gland. As an agent that 'electrocutes' or attacks invader organisms, copper prevents infection by viruses attempting to invade the body. Dispatched by the spleen, copper works as part of the auto-immune and excretory systems. Copper is required for the absorption of iron and the formation of red cells. Copper checks and balances the transport of iron which in turn regulates oxygen transport. The major antagonist of copper is zinc. High levels of copper have been known to cause severe mental upset. Dr Carl Pfeiffer pioneered his work in using zinc to reduce levels of copper and spermine. Copper works directly with tyrosine regulating enzyme and energy producers, from the thyroid and adrenal glands. Copper is a highly toxic micro-nutrient when excessive. Mood swings and mental disturbances accompany toxic amounts of copper. High copper levels will increase cholesterol in the blood and cause a build up of calcium in the veins and arteries. The skin, hair, liver, brain and kidney have high amounts of deposited copper.

Oysters, liver, lentils, parsley, walnuts, bread, watercress and lean meats all contain copper. High amounts of copper have found their way into the food chain from processed food additives, piped contaminated water, pesticides, herbicides and fertilisers etc.

There is no RDA in the UK. In the USA, the RDA is 2.0–3.0mg. Copper should only be given therapeutically under careful chemical analysis and scrutiny.

Fluoride has a close working relationship with calcium and silica; it assists the absorption and utilisation of calcium and prevents an excess of calcium in the gut. Fluoride gives bones and teeth their shine. It also has antiseptic qualities.

Joint pains, toothache, joint troubles, may suggest an imbalance of fluoride.

Oats, sunflower seeds, garlic, green vegetables, almonds and sea vegetables are high in fluoride.

No RDA has been set. Adults: 1–4mg.

Iodine is a major regulator of the thyroid gland. The thyroid's connection with the pituitary as the master controller of the body is affected by iodine. The thyroid controls the metabolism of food and iodine helps ignite the release of energy from food. Weight, energy and emotional feelings are all dramatically affected by low iodine levels. Low iodine will cause lethargy, fatigue, skin troubles, eczema, low libido, reduced blood pressure and may cause anaemia. Depression, anxiety and fear are all symptoms of low iodine, as is goitre, an enlargement of the thyroid.

Most seafoods are high in iodine. The best source of iodine is dulse, a sea vegetable.

The use of radioactive iodine in patients with thyroid trouble causes poisoning. Iodine needs calcium and phosphorus to balance it and keep it 'under control'.

The UK RDA is 140mcg. Under strict monitoring, doses of up to 2mg are safe.

Iron is the most important oxygen transporter in the bloodstream. It is essential to muscle tissues and is an important link in the process of freeing oxygen from the breath and energy from food. Iron is absorbed in the duodenum and jejunum via the intestinal mucosa, and stored in the liver, spleen and bone marrow.

Iron is depressed by vitamin C. Deficiencies of iron cause anaemia, immune problems, lethargy, depression. Apricots, peaches, prunes, raisins, yeast, whole grains, watercress, mustard and cress, meats, spinach, beetroot, lentils and sesame seeds are all high in iron.

The UK RDA is 12mg.

Magnesium helps keep acidity levels down. It is necessary for the conversion of food into energy and important for the absorption and utilisation of all proteins, fats and carbohydrates. Magnesium is an important mineral for the healthy transmission of signals from nerves to muscles. Magnesium works with calcium in the balance of acid and alkaline. Along with potassium

and phosphorus, these are by far the most important minerals
for a healthy body, mind and spirit.

When the magnesium levels drop, energy falls, toxic waste
builds up, the impact of stress on the nervous system increases
and takes its toll. Muscle weakness, fatigue, lethargy, blood
sugar troubles (characterised by low energy in the day and too
much mental energy at night, which leads to sleeplessness) can
all develop from a deficiency.

All nuts and seeds contain magnesium, as do legumes
(especially lentils), sea vegetables and all green leafy vegetables, especially watercress, and mustard and cress.

Manganese   acts as 'fuel distributor' in the blood and as a nerve
and muscle stabiliser. It is also important for the synthesis of DNA
and RNA. Manganese reduces the impact of stress on the myelin
sheath that coats the nerves and all the nerve pathways by
reducing the 'electricity' of the nervous system. It is essential to
the healing of any damage, sprain, strain or other injury to the
skeletal muscular system. In large amounts of vitamins C, B5, B1
and calcium and magnesium, manganese will act as an anti-
spasmodic and as a natural painkiller.

Cereals, grains, beans, meats, fish, eggs and leafy greens are
all high in manganese.

There is no UK RDA. By US standards a RDA would be
2–6mg. For any acute pain take 30–40mg; for chronic pain 25mg
every 4–6 hours can be helpful. It is recommended to stop using
it for 1 week after 3 or 4 weeks' treatment.

Phosphorus   works with calcium to maintain the acid-alkaline
balance and move the body back towards the carbon side of the
carbon-nitrogen cycle. An essential component of bones and
teeth, phosphorus also works hard at the energy conversion of
fats and protein and the associated metabolic processes. All
foods contain phosphorus and so it is virtually impossible to
have a deficiency of this substance. If too much phosphorus
shows up in the blood it indicates the movement towards

over-acidity and will begin to create calcium deposits in the veins, arteries and vital organs. Where there is too much phosphorus there will be too much calcium. High levels of phosphorus in the blood reveals 'food additive' poisoning and processed food 'trauma'.

The UK RDA is 800mg, all of which can be derived from food sources. Taking supplements of phosphorus is never indicated apart from as a tissue salt, prescribed by a practitioner.

Potassium   As the major 'salt' balance mineral, potassium works to keep vital fluids circulating through the blood and all tissue, as a 'bath of life'. Every cell requires constant and fresh supplies of potassium for its energy to flow. Potassium is one of the main regulating minerals for the acid-alkaline balance of all the bodily fluids. Potassium helps create the 'movement' of the muscles, nerves and cell life of the body and affects its motion, activity and endurance. Potassium is vital to the heart and heart rhythms. It regulates the elimination of waste to and through the kidneys, via the heart and circulation. It literally 'pushes' waste through the body.

All strong stimulants, as well as environmental toxins, affect the movement and flow of potassium, reducing the overall energy (electricity) of the body. When under stress the body uses greater amounts of potassium to enable emergency alert (fight or flight) response.

Potassium salts are the quickest to get into the bloodstream and are needed during periods of dehydration. Many of the popular salts (electrolytes) for fluid replacement contain too much sugar. They are to be avoided. Lemon water with sea salt, orange juice with some unsweetened white or red grape juice is much better for preventing dehydration after exercise. All vegetables contain potassium. Celery, parsley, carrots, watercress, leafy greens, bananas, sunflower seeds and all nuts and seeds are good sources.

RDA in the UK is not established. By conservative estimates the body needs 1,900–6,500mg of potassium, depending on levels of activity and stress. The optimum form of supplemented potassium is potassium citrate. Many food additives and preservatives contain high amounts of potassium-based compounds to prevent fats from becoming rancid.

Selenium works closely with vitamin E as an anti-oxidant, preventing the build up of free radicals. It also helps support the transport of oxygen to the cell via haemoglobin. In so doing it helps reduce cell level acidity and increases the move towards alkalinity. Because of this function it may help to slow down and possibly reverse the ageing process. Selenium protects cellular membranes. It may also be helpful to the liver, restoring enzyme activity and the purification of blood. Along with the amino acid methionine, selenium scans the body for 'energy thieves' that rob the blood of its 2 most precious substances, sugar and oxygen.

Unless there is specific evidence to suggest higher, regular amounts, be careful with selenium. It is a powerful substance that works in subtle ways. Derived from the Greek word for moon, it was believed that selenium affected emotional ups and downs. High doses tend to affect moods. High amounts of selenium can cause skin disturbances by increasing the activity of sulphur. Low selenium levels in the soil are known to increase the risk of cancer and therefore must be supplemented in the dietary intake.

Grains, cheese, almonds and nuts, fish and seafoods contain selenium. As a supplement, selenium should be taken in small doses. Selenium supplements have been successfully marketed, heralded as the panacea for cancer. However, the need for selenium depends on many things, and too much selenium is dangerous. Too much can disturb the balance of the other minerals.

No RDA exists in the UK. A dose of 100mcg taken regularly is suggested. Only in selenomethionine form can supplements be properly absorbed through the gut.

Silica works closely with sodium, potassium, calcium and iron, thereby affecting every system in the body. With calcium, silica supports the bones and muscles. With potassium and phosphorus, silica maintains the bodily fluids. With calcium and magnesium, silica plays a role in the acid-alkaline cycle. With copper, silica aids the transport of oxygen and prevents waste getting back into the cells. If the food balance of fats, proteins and carbohydrates is not right, supplemented forms of silica will be thrown out by the body.

There is no RDA for silica. Supplementation should be taken in herbal form as horsetail herb, Kervan Silica, or homeopathic silica.

Sodium is essential for 'holding' the other minerals in check. Sodium maintains the correct acidity level in the vital fluids such as saliva, urine and blood. The movement of sodium is synonymous with the movement of water and fluids. When there is too much acidity, sodium is required to restore balance, but an increase of sodium can harden the soft tissue of the body.

Moderate salt should be taken in the summertime, less in the winter months.

Cheese, vegetables, celery, leafy greens, beetroots, carrots, grains, yoghurt and fish all contain sodium. The forms of sodium used in processed foods are harmful to the liver and kidneys.

There is no RDA. The body requires more than 2,000mg of sodium every day to function. Sodium chloride (table salt) is harmful to the body because it causes too much fluid to build up inside the body. Magnesium chloride or sea salt is much better.

Zinc is the most important micro-nutrient for the immune system, particularly the thymus gland. Zinc also plays a vital role in the proper functioning of the adrenal glands. Adrenals help regulate the energy conversion cycle, and the hormones for energy and stress. Zinc has long been associated with 'virility' and male potency. It is also important for the prostate.

All seafoods, all sea vegetables, sesame seeds and pumpkin
seeds contain zinc.

The RDA is not established in the UK. In the USA, the RDA
is 15mg. Optimal doses are 30–75mg per day.

Vanadium   Until recently vanadium was only known for its
antagonistic role to fat and cholesterol. More specifically,
vanadium plays a vital role as an 'adjuster' micro-nutrient for the
respiratory system. Vanadium helps the utilisation of oxygen
and the elimination of carbon dioxide in the process of breathing. This is its main function, joining forces with oxygen to make
a 'pushing' force for utilisation of oxygen, particularly during an
emergency when energy demands in the body are greater.

No RDA exists.

Specific Illness
Reference List

Abscess   Infection with pus in any body part   *Group 1*

Acne   Skin disorders – pimples, whiteheads, blackheads on back, face, shoulders, chest, arm   *Group 19*

Adrenal exhaustion   A reduction of the stress 'fight or flight' mechanism leading to depletion of vital secretions   *Group 13*

Allergies   A sensitivity to a particular substance that cannot be pushed away or neutralised   *Group 23*

Anaemia   A reduced amount of any red blood cell-forming materials   *Group 20*

Arteriosclerosis   A hardening of the walls of the arteries or vital organs   *Groups 11 and 22*

Arthritis   Inflammation/infection of the joints leading to an inability to produce antibodies that distinguish healthy cells   *Group 22*

Asthma   An acute/chronic respiratory disorder causing choking, suffocation, wheezing, inability to breathe   *Group 23*

Backache   A general weakness of ligaments and muscles causing pain and strains   *Group 9*

Baldness   and hair loss   *Groups 1 and 17/18*

Bronchitis   Inflammation of air passages leading to weakness of lungs   *Groups 7, 5 and 1*

Cancer   An unhealthy, unnatural division of immature cells decaying and affecting the surrounding tissue   *Group 1*

Cataracts   The eye lens becomes clouded – opaque   *Group 20*

Coeliac disease   A disorder caused by inability to process gluten from wheat, rye and barley leading to irritation of the intestinal tract   *Group 3*

Cholesterol   (High) Unusually high blood lipid (fat) content *Groups 2 and 11*

Cirrhosis of the liver   Degeneration of liver cells due to alcohol, viral bacteria invasion   *Group 6*

Cold   Inflammation of ears, nose, throat, sinus and increased catarrh   *Group 1*

Colitis   Inflammation of mucous membrane of the bowel, colon, large intestine   *Group 3*

Constipation   Disorder of bowel elimination resulting in blockage, inability to defecate   *Group 3*

Cystic fibrosis   Hereditary disease affecting many glands and organs. Thick mucus promotes bacterial growth   *Group 1*

Cystitis   Inflammation of urinary tract affecting kidneys and bladder   *Group 16*

Dermatitis   Inflammatory skin reaction producing several types of skin troubles   *Group 19*

Diarrhoea   Frequent elimination, cramps, spasm and dehydration   *Group 3*

Diabetes   A metabolic imbalance of the pancreas. Inability to manufacture insulin and utilise carbohydrates   *Groups 6 and 20*

Diverticulitis   Inflammation of the small sacs in the colon, making it difficult to empty the bowel efficiently   *Group 20*

Dizziness   A sensation of extreme random motion sickness *Group 10*

Eczema   Skin inflammation, itchy, scaly redness   *Group 19*

Emphysema   A degenerative lung disorder leading to inability to breathe properly   *Groups 1, 5 and 7*

Epilepsy   A disease causing seizure due to imbalanced neurological brain activity   *Group 14*

Fatigue   Feeling physical or mental exhaustion   *Group 13*

Flatulence   Digestive disorder from improperly processing food   *Group 4*

Fever   Abnormal elevation of body temperature above 99°F   *Group 1*

Flu An acute viral infection of the respiratory tract *Groups 1 and 7*

Gastro intestinal flu *Groups 1 and 3*

Gall bladder Inadequate supply of bile causes hard stools and other symptoms *Group 6*

Gastritis Inflammation of mucous membrane of stomach lining *Group 4*

Goitre Enlargement of the thyroid due to hormone imbalance *Group 10*

Gout High uric acid build up due to toxins *Group 9*

Halitosis Bad breath caused by digestive and bowel troubles. Teeth and gum infections *Groups 3 and 4*

Hay fever Reaction to pollens, causing inflammation of eyes, ears, nose, throat *Group 23*

Headaches Tension, pressure, pain in any part of the head *Group 14*

Heart disease Weakening of the chief muscle that runs the circulatory system *Group 2*

Haemophilia A lack of blood clotting agents, causing prolonged bleeding and bruising *Groups 10 and 11*

Hepatitis Inflammation due to toxic substances congesting the liver *Group 6*

Herpes A virus – chickenpox, shingles or sexually transmitted *Groups 1 and 19*

Hyperactivity Disorder of the central nervous system causing abnormal aggressive, impulsive behavourial problems, sleep disturbances *Group 12*

Hypertension High blood pressure *Groups 2 and 11*

Hyperthyroidism Over-production of hormones by the thyroid gland *Group 10*

Hypoglycaemia Abnormally variable high/low blood sugar affecting absorption and assimilation of foods *Groups 13 and 20*

Hypotension Low blood pressure causing lethargy and low oxygen availability to tissue *Groups 11 and 13*

Hypothyroidism Underproduction of thyroid hormones

resulting in extremely low metabolism   *Group 10*

Indigestion   Discomfort before or after eating due to high acidity or alkalinity   *Group 4*

Infection   An elevated white cell reaction due to bacterial or viral invasion   *Group 1*

Irritable bowel   Inflammation causing soreness in any part of the bowel or intestine   *Group 3*

Kidney diseases   Any disruption, inflammation, infection of the nephron ducts or inability to eliminate wastes   *Group 16*

Jaundice   A yellowish taint of the skin and eyes resulting from worn-out red cells   *Group 6*

Meningitis   Infection of the membranes between the skull and brain. Bacterial, viral or fungal   *Groups 1 and 12*

Multiple Sclerosis   A chronic disease causing degeneration of the myelin coating of the nerves   *Groups 4 and 12*

Muscular Dystrophy   A progressive disease to the muscle–nerve–brain communication   *Groups 9, 12 and 13*

Myasthenia   A loss of transmission of the nerve impulse   *Groups 12, 13 and 14*

Nausea   An over-alkaline condition in the stomach/bowel   *Groups 1 and 21*

Neuritis   Inflammation of any nerve or nerve pathway   *Groups 1 and 12*

Oedema   Fluid retention caused by excessive acidity   *Group 21*

Osteoporosis   A reduction of size and mass of bone density   *Groups 1 and 22*

Obesity   An increase of 20 per cent body weight   *Groups 14 and 17/18*

Pancreatitis   Inflammation of the pancreas inhibiting insulin production   *Groups 1 and 20*

Parkinson's Disease   A disease in which the nerves degenerate   *Groups 12, 13, 14 and 17/18*

Pneumonia   Inflammation/infection of the lungs creating mucus   *Groups 1, 19 and 23*

Prostatitis   Inflammation of the prostate causing burning, calculi, blood, pus, frequency of urination *Groups 1 and 16*

Psoriasis A skin disease causing recurring skin patches and scales anywhere on the body *Groups 1, 15 and 19*

Pyorrhea Infected gum or tooth disease with pus, blood, loosening of teeth *Groups 1, 11 and 22*

Rheumatism General acute/chronic stiffness of muscles and pain in joints *Groups 1, 9 and 22*

Rhinitis Inflammation of nasal passage and membrane *Group 5*

Sciatica Severe muscle nerve pain travelling down the back of the thigh *Groups 1, 9 and 12*

Shingles see *Herpes*

Sinusitis Inflammation of sinus cavities causing excess catarrh *Groups 1 and 5*

Stroke A cerebral and circulatory breakdown of an area of the brain cells *Groups 1, 14 and 17/18*

Tonsillitis Swelling and increased concentration of poisons in the tonsils causing inflammation infection *Groups 1 and 5*

Tuberculosis A contagious bacterial infection of the lungs *Groups 1, 17/18, 19 and 23*

Vaginitis A burning soreness of the vulva and the vaginal opening *Groups 1, 16 and 19*

Venereal disease Sexually transmitted diseases such as Gonorrhea, syphilis, chlamydia *Groups 1, 8 and 17/18*

Resource Guide

GROUP 1
Solgar B complex with C tablet
Bio-care liquid B-complex
Bio-care capsule B-complex
Solgar pantothenic acid 200mg tablet
Solgar pantothenic acid 550mg capsule

GROUP 2
Solgar Vite 400i.u. succinate
Bio-care vite 300i.u.
Solgar CoQ10 30 or 60mg

GROUP 3
Solgar VN-2,000 tablet
Solgar multi-II capsule
Bio-care multi vitamin mineral capsule
Calcium ascorbate Solgar
Magnesium ascorbate Bio-care
Solgar digestive enzyme
Bio-care digest aid
Solgar dadelion, golden seal, aloe vera (herb capsules)
Solgar chelated calcium
Solgar chelated magnesium
Bio-care ligazyme
Bio-care liquid B-complex

GROUP 4
Solgar acidophilus with bifidus
Bio-care acidophilus

Bio-care digest-aid
Solgar digestive enzyme
Nelson biochemic tissue salt mag. phos.
Bio-care ligazyme
Solgar Pantothenic acid
Nelson biochemic tissue salt ferr. phos.

GROUP 5
Calcium ascorbate Solgar 500mg
Magnesium ascorbate Bio-care 500mg
Solgar beta carotene
Bio-care liquid vit. A
Solgar dry vit. E succinate
Bio-care 300i.u. vit. E
Biofore Echinaforce echinacea
Ortis propolis spray

GROUP 6
Bio-care Oxyplex
Bio-care ligazyme
Solgar phosphatidyl choline
Green Magma
Solgar digestive betaine hydrochloride
Seredyn ginko biloba
Solgar ginko biloba
Solgar gota kola
Solgar antioxidants formula
Bio-care HEP-194
Bio-care Cellguard

GROUP 7
Multi-mineral Bio-care Complex
Aspartamins Solgar
Solgar Yerba Santa capsules
Solgar mullein capsules

GROUP 8
Solgar VM-2,000
Solgar Multi II capsules
Bio-care multi vitamin mineral
Solgar Dong Quai
Bio-care calcium EAP
Bio-care ligazyme
Solgar pyridoxal-5-phosphate B-6
Bio-care magnesium EAP
Bio-care mega GLA
Solgar ginseng capsules

GROUP 9
Solgar VM-2,000
Solgar Multi II capsules
Bio-care multi vitamin mineral
Solgar calcium ascorbate
Bio-care magnesium ascorbate
Solgar pantothenic acid
Bio-care calcium EAP
Bio-care magnesium EAP
Bio-care digest-aid

GROUP 10
Solgar Aspartamins
Bio-care multimineral complex
Solgar kelp tablets
Calcium ascorbate Solgar
Magnesium ascorbate Bio-care
Solgar B2
Solgar niacin No-Flush
Nelson Homeopathic Lycopodium 6

GROUP 11
Solgar calcium ascorbate
Solgar Bioflavonoids

Solgar No-Flush niacin
Solgar calcium ascorbate
Bio-care magnesium ascorbate
Solgar Rutin

GROUP 12
Bio-care B-complex
Solgar B-complex
Bio-care calcium EAP
Bio-care magnesium EAP
Bio-care NT-188

GROUP 13
Solgar pantothenic acid
Bio-care AD-206

GROUP 14
Solgar Multi II capsules
Solgar VM-2,000
Bio-care multi vitamin mineral
Bio-care NT-188
Bio-care mineral complex
Solgar Aspartamin
Solgar Neuro-nutrients

GROUP 15
Spirulina Lifestream Ltd
Solgar calcium ascorbate
Bio-care magnesium ascorbate

GROUP 16
Solgar Uva Ursi capsules
Ainsworth Homeopath Pharmacy
Sabal Surrealetta 6c or 30c

GROUPS 17 and 18
Solgar Multi II capsules
Solgar VM-2,000
Bio-care multi vitamin mineral
Solgar Ginseng
Bio-care vit. E 300i.u.
Solgar vit. E dry form succinate
Solgar tyrosine

GROUP 19
Solgar Multi II capsules
Solgar VM-2,000
Bio-care multi vitamin mineral capsules
Bio-care liquid vit. A

GROUP 20
Bio-liquid chromium
Solgar GTF chromium picolinate
Bio-care multi mineral complex

GROUP 21
Nelson homeopathic nat. mur. (homeopathic salt) 6
Bio-care Mega GIA
Gerard House Agnus Castus

GROUP 22
Solgar Aspartamins
Bio-care multi mineral
Bio-care Ligazyme
Nelson homeopathic tissue salts:
    Calc. phos. (calcium phosphate)
    Calc. sulp. (calcium sulphate)

GROUP 23
Solgar zinc picolinate
Bio-care zinc citrate

Bio-care B-complex
Solgar B-complex
Solgar pantothenic acid
Solgar calcium ascorbate
Bio-care magnesium ascorbate

GROUP 24
Solgar calcium ascorbate
Bio-care magnesium ascorbate
Solgar B-complex
Bio-care B-complex
Bio-care B12
Solgar B12
Solgar Aspartamins
Bio-care multimineral complex

The products listed in this resource guide can be purchased at leading health-food stores and chemists or by contacting them direct:

Ainsworth Homeopathic Pharmacy
38 New Cavendish Street
London W1M 4RH   071 935 5330

Bio-Care
54 Northfield Road
Kings Norton, Birmingham
B30 1JH, UK   021 433 3727

Gerard House Ltd
475 Capability Green
Luton, Bedfordshire
LU1 3LU   0582 487331

Ivano Fruiterer
44 Tachbrook Street
London SW1   071 834 1850

Lifestream
Ash House, Stedham
Midhurst, W. Sussex
GU29 0PT   0730 813642

Nelson Pharmacy
73 Duke Street
London W1

Ortis Company   0992 575162

Dr Reckeweg
Complex Homeopathy
19 Park Street
Bolton
BL1 4BD   0204 384 550
          Fax 0204 384 844

Solgar Vitamins Ltd
Solgar House
Chiltern Commerce Centre
Chesham, Bucks
HP5 2PY   0494 791691

Vitalia-Paradise
Kneip
Hemel Hempstead, Herts
HP2 4TF   0442 231 155

Weleda UK Ltd
Heanor Road
Ilkeston
Derbyshire DE7 8DR

Bibliography

Airola, Paavlo Dr, *Are You Confused*, Foreword by Leslie H. Salov M.D., (Phoenix, Arizona, Health Plus Publishers, 1971)

Ibid., *Every Woman's Book*, Foreword by Mary Ann Kibler, M.D., Introduction by Robert S. Mendelsohn, M.D. (Phoenix, Arizona, Health Plus Publishers, 1979)

Ibid., *How to Get Well*, Forword by H. Rudolph Alsleben, M.D., Medical eds H. Rudolph Alsleben, M.D., Barnet Meltzer, M.D., Alan Nittler M.D. (Phoenix, Arizona, Health Plus Publishers, 1974)

Atkins, Robert C. Dr *Dr Atkins' Nutrition Breakthrough*, (New York, Bantam Books, 1981)

Bieler, Henry G., *Food is Your Best Medicine*, (New York, Random House, 1965)

Borsaak, Henry, *Vitamins*, (New York, Pyramid Books, 1940)

Bosco, Dominick & Rosenbaum, Michael E. M.D., *The Super Supplement Bible*, (Wellingborough, Northamptonshire, Thorson Publishing Group Ltd, 1988)

Boericke, William, *Pocket Manual of Homeopathic Materia Medica, Comprising the Characteristic and Guiding Symptoms of all Remedies*, (Philadelphia, USA, Boericke and Runyon, Boericke and Tafel Inc., 1927)

Braverman, Eric, R., M.D. with Carl C. Pfeiffer M.D., PhD., *The Healing Nutrients Within. Facts Finding and New Research on Amino Acids*, (New Canaan, Connecticut, Keats Publishing Inc., 1987)

Clark, John, Henry M.D., *A Dictionary of Practical Materia Medica*, (3 vols, New Delhi, India, Health Science Press, Jain Publishing Company, 1978)

Clark, John, Henry, *The Prescriber*, (8th edn, Rushington, England, Health Science Press, 1968)

Clark, Linda, *Get Well Naturally*, (New York, Devin-Adair Co., 1965)

Davis, Adelle, *Let's Get Well*, (New York, Harcourt Brace and World, 1965; New York, New American Library, 1972)

Ibid. and Marshall Mandell, *Let's Have Healthy Children*, (New York, New American Library, 1979)

Dossey, Larry, Dr M.D., *Healing Breakthroughs, How your Attitudes and Beliefs can Affect Your Health*, (London, Piatkus Publishers, 1991)

Ibid., *Space, Time and Medicine*, Foreword by Fritjof Capra, (Boston and London, New Science Library, Shambhala, 1982)

Garvey, John W. J.R. *The Five Phases of Foods*, vol. 1. (Mass., Well-Being Books, 1982)

Earle, Liz, *Vital Oils*, (London, Ebury Press, 1991)

Lust, John, N.D., DBM, *The Herb Book*, (Bantam Books, 1974)

Jouanny, Jacques, *The Essentials of Homeopathic Therapeutics*, (Delmas Bordeaux 2000-1-80 France, Laboratories Boiron, 1980)

Kaptchuk, Ted. J. OMD, *The Web That Has No Weaver*, (New York City, Congdon and Weed, 1983)

Kloss, Jethro, *Back to Eden*, (New York, Beneficial Books, 1972)

Lewis-Elvin, Lewis Walter H., *Medical Botany Plants Affecting Man's Health*, (New York, John Wiley & Sons, 1977)

Lappé Frances Moore, *Diet for a Small Planet*, 10th Anniversary edn, (Toronto, Canada, Ballantine Books, Random House of Canada, 1982)

Muramoto, Naboru, *Healing Ourselves*, Ed. Michael Abehsera., (New York, Avon Books, 1973)

Merck, Manual, *Diagnosis and Therapy*, 15th edn, Robert Berkow, M.D., Fletcher Andrew J. M.B., B.Chir., Assistant Ed, (Merck Sharp & Dohme Research Laboratories, 1987)

Null, Gary & Steve Null, *The Complete Handbook of Nutrition*, (New York, Robert Speller and Sons, 1972)

Nutrition Almanac, 2nd edn, (Minneapolis, Minn, Nutrition Search, 1973)

Peletier, Kenneth, R. *Holistic Medicine, From Stress to Optimum Health*, Introduction by Norman Cousins, (New York, Delta/Seymour Lawrence Ed., A Merloyd Lawrence Book. Dell Publishing Co. Inc. 1979)

Ibid., *Toward a Science of Consciousness*, (Berkeley, California, Celestial Arts, 1985)

Pfeiffer, Carl C. *Mental and Elemental Nutrients*, (New Canaan, Conn., Keats Publishing, 1980)

Reckeweg-Homeopathic Specialties: Pharmazeutische Vols. 1 & 2, Fabrik, Dr Reckeweg & Co GmbH Bensheim, Germany.

Recommended Dietary Allowances, 9th edn, (Washington D.C., National Academy of Sciences, 1980)

Royal, Penny C., *Herbally Yours*, (Utah, USA, BiWorld Publishers Inc., 1979)

Rogers, Carl. R., *A Way of Being*, (Boston, Mass, Houghton Mifflin Company, 1980)

Scogna, Joseph, *The Promethion Life Energy Foundation* (1980)

Shute, Wilfred E. & Harold Taub, *Vitamin E for Ailing and Healthy Hearts*, (New York, Pyramid House, 1969)

Veith, Ilza, *The Yellow Emperor's Classic Manual of Internal Medicine*, (London, England, University of California Press Ltd., 1972)

Wade, Carlson, *Helping Your Health With Enzymes*, (New York, Universal-Award House, 1971)

Williams, Roger J. *Nutrition Against Disease*, (New York, Pitman Publ., 1971)

Ibid., & Dwight K. Kalita, eds. *A Physician's Handbook on Orthomolecular Medicine*, (New Canaan, Conn., Keats Publishing, 1977)

Woodward, Robert. *Better Health: A Practical Guide to Some Nutritional and Alternative Approaches*, (Southsea, Errand Press Ltd., 1988)